Look Great

Advance Praise for *Look Great, Live Green*

"I don't have many 'can't-live-without' products, but Sumbody's Lucky Lips Lip Balm is one of them. Deborah has masterfully combined supereffective potions with adorable packaging, and the entire line is genius. And I had a wonderful time at the Sumbody store and Sumtime Spa—it was amazing, even for a jaded beauty editor!"

— Chloe Redmond Warner
San Francisco Editor,
Lucky magazine

"Using truly natural and toxin-free products is so important in a spa environment, and our search for the cleanest products available led us to Deborah Burnes and Sumbody. I have yet to meet someone as educated and passionate about using the purest ingredients nature has to offer and using them in the ways they best benefit the skin and body. Deborah has taught me and my staff so much about ingredients, preservative systems, and harmful synthetics and chemicals. In an industry that is difficult to decipher at times, we now feel confident and armed with the knowledge and products that are safe for our clients, who are increasingly concerned about the safety of skin- and body-care products."

— Jeannie Jarnot
Director of Spa and Retail Operations
The Carneros Inn, a PlumpJack Resort

Ordering

Trade bookstores in the U.S. and Canada please contact:

Publishers Group West
1700 Fourth Street, Berkeley CA 94710
Phone: (800) 788-3123   Fax: (800) 351-5073

Hunter House books are available at bulk discounts for
textbook course adoptions; to qualifying community, health-care,
and government organizations; and for special promotions and
fund-raising. For details please contact:

Special Sales Department
Hunter House Inc., PO Box 2914, Alameda CA 94501-0914
Phone: (510) 865-5282   Fax: (510) 865-4295
E-mail: ordering@hunterhouse.com

Individuals can order our books from most bookstores,
by calling (**800**) **266-5592**, or from our website at
www.hunterhouse.com

Look Great,
Live Green

Choosing Beauty Solutions
That Are Planet-Safe
and Budget-Smart

Deborah Burnes

Hunter House
PUBLISHERS

Hunter House Inc., Publishers
PO Box 2914
Alameda CA 94501-0914

Library of Congress Cataloging-in-Publication Data
Burnes, Deborah.
Look great, live green : choosing beauty solutions that are planet-safe and budget-smart / Deborah Burnes. — 1st ed.
p.   cm.
Includes bibliographical references and index.
ISBN 978-0-89793-521-0 (pbk. : alk. paper)
1. Hygiene products—Environmental aspects.   2. Cosmetics—Environmental aspects.   3. Beauty, Personal.   I. Title.
RA778.5.B87 2009
613'.4—dc22   2009024379

Project Credits
Cover Design: Brian Dittmar Graphic Design
Book Production: John McKercher
Copy Editor: Margaret Wimberger
Proofreader: John David Marion
Indexer: Nancy D. Peterson
Editor: Alexandra Mummery
Editorial Intern: Ashley Zeal
Production Intern: Sara Hamling
Senior Marketing Associate: Reina Santana
Publicity Associate: Sean Harvey
Rights Coordinator: Candace Groskreutz
Customer Service Manager: Christina Sverdrup
Order Fulfillment: Washul Lakdhon
Administrator: Theresa Nelson
Computer Support: Peter Eichelberger
Publisher: Kiran S. Rana

Printed and bound by Bang Printing, Brainerd, Minnesota

Manufactured in the United States of America

9 8 7 6 5 4 3 2 1   First Edition   09 10 11 12 13

Contents

PART II: Let's Go Comparison Shopping

Foreword

by Frank Lipman, MD

As a physician trained in Western medicine, I was taught to make a diagnosis or name the disease, and then prescribe a treatment. But as I gained experience, I began to realize that this "name-it, blame-it, and tame-it" approach was not effective because it failed to deal with the root causes of my patients' illnesses. I found myself continually asking, "Isn't there a better way?" And, more importantly, "How can I help my patients prevent illness in the first place?"

As the founder of Eleven Eleven Wellness Center in New York City, I've spent the better part of my career carefully developing a progressive approach to health care by combining both Western and Eastern medicines with other therapies to practice what is now being called *Integrative Medicine*. Simply put, I've taken my formal education; augmented it with years of intensive research that incorporates acupuncture, herbs, yoga, diet, nutrition, stress reduction, vitamins, and detoxification; and combined them into a medical and healing practice. I'm now able to use this healthy, natural, and comprehensive modality to address my patients' needs without having to resort to drugs and surgery.

From Chinese medicine I have learned that we humans are a microcosm of a great macrocosm: the planet earth. Therefore, hand in hand with the goal of a healthier self, we need to be conscious of the state of our precious earth. So how do we—already overwhelmed with news and information—integrate the core principles of our own health with the needs of the planet?

It was while doing research for my own two books on health, *Total Renewal* and *Spent*, that I became acutely aware of the dangers lurking inside our bathroom cabinets and cosmetics bags. I was surprised to discover that the use of common personal-care products exposed the average American to more than one-hundred different chemicals each day. Then in 2004, a more shocking truth revealed itself to me when the results of a study on these products was released by the nonprofit Environmental Working Group (EWG). The EWG compared about 10,000 ingredients found in 7,500 different products against lists of known or suspected chemical health hazards. Incredibly, of the 7,500 products tested by the EWG, nearly one-third contained ingredients classified as possible carcinogens. Yet of those 7,500 products, only 28 had ever been evaluated for safety by the Cosmetic Ingredient Review panel (CIR). And while the cosmetic industry asserts that their products are safe, 89 percent of the ingredients used in cosmetics today have not been assessed by either the FDA or the industry itself.

So who's looking out for us? Although most people assume that the FDA oversees the cosmetics industry, it actually has very little power when it comes to regulating the ingredients found in beauty products. Except for color additives and a few widely prohibited substances, manufacturers may use any ingredient or raw material to create a personal-care product without any government review or approval whatsoever. In scenarios all-too-reminiscent of the era when industry-paid scientists denied that smoking caused cancer, or, more recently, when oil lobbyists denied the existence of global warming, the cosmetics industry claims its products are safe, but the testing, monitoring, and oversight of these claims is left in the hands of the very scientists these companies employ to do that testing.

The rest of the world isn't turning a blind eye, however. And so far, the Europeans are taking this much more seriously than we are in the United States. In 2005 a directive passed in the European Union mandating that chemicals determined to be carcinogens, mutagens, or reproductive toxins must be removed from cosmetics sold there. Interestingly, most countries throughout the world, including China, are following the European Union's lead.

But too scant attention has been paid to this topic domestically, where laws similar to those passed in the European Union have yet to be adopted. In America, we are told that chemicals are innocent until proven guilty, that there are "acceptable" levels of contamination our bodies can tolerate, and that a certain amount of pollution and disease is the price we pay for modern life.

But is there a middle ground? And if not, what is the *real* price for all of this?

In terms of increased health-care costs, rising rates of cancer and infertility, as well as an explosion in learning disabilities in our children, the cost of our head-in-the-sand approach is incalculable. Add to that the new science of epigenetics, which is proving that the damage done to our genes by these toxins is being passed onto the next generation, and I don't believe I'm being overly dramatic when I say that we are playing Russian roulette with our future.

So how do we fight back? And what can be done to help us heal ourselves, our children, and the planet? The cosmetics industry is a $60 billion a-year goliath that doesn't want you to know the truth about its products. But information is power, and in *Look Great, Live Green* Deborah Burnes provides us with everything we need to know to make better personal-care product choices. With an insider's view and nerves of steel, Deborah goes right after the monster. She not only reveals the *true* origins of some of the most popular brands of cosmetics—where and how they're *really* made—she also outlines a detailed program we can all follow to make ourselves and, in the process, our precious planet, more healthy. She provides advice on adopting simpler habits and making smarter consumer choices, such as selecting personal-care products with more than one use. Organic shampoo as soap? Olive oil to remove makeup? Both offer a fraction of the environmental and health impacts of popular mainstream products.

Of course, all of this means that selecting natural personal-care products is urgent, but it can also be easy *and* fun. What makes *Look Great, Live Green* so wonderful but also so simple is the incredible amount of passion Deborah Burnes has for our health and the environment. Having seen the dark side of the cosmetics industry, she has chosen to walk the walk of "going green" in her daily life; in the founding and running of her own company, Sumbody Skin Care;

and, most importantly, as a mother. She does as she says! And so should we.

Read and learn from *Look Great, Live Green*. The result will be improved health and beauty for you and your family and a better, cleaner planet for all to enjoy.

— Frank Lipman, MD
Founder and director of the Eleven Eleven
Wellness Center in NY
Author of *Spent; End Exhaustion and Feel Great Again*;
and *Total Renewal: Seven Key Steps to Resilience,
Vitality and Long-Term Health*

Important Note

The material in this book is intended to provide a review of information regarding body-care products and skin health. Every effort has been made to provide accurate and dependable information. The contents of this book have been compiled through professional research and in consultation with medical and health professionals. However, health-care professionals have differing opinions, and advances in medical and scientific research are made very quickly, so some of the information may become outdated.

Therefore, the publisher, authors, and editors, as well as the professionals quoted in the book, cannot be held responsible for any error, omission, or dated material. The authors and publisher assume no responsibility for any outcome of applying the information in this book in a program of self-care or under the care of a licensed practitioner. If you have questions concerning your skin or health, or about the application of the information described in this book, consult a qualified health-care professional.

Acknowledgments

Writing this book was an unexpected inspiration to me. I want to create a public awareness about the potential harmful effects the beauty industry can have on our health and environment. I want to educate consumers so they can make choices that are in-line with their comfort levels of exposure. It is important to me to offer solutions. I did not want just another "we-are-all-doomed-and-killing-ourselves-and-our-families-daily" type of book. It is not how I see the situation. Rather I believe once we are aware, we can make change happen. Once we know, we can see what we need to do. Knowledge is power, and armed with the proper information, we can have a brighter future. This book was an unexpected inspiration to me, because I was fortunate enough to get a glimpse at this brighter future while writing it. The level of support and the qualities of the people who helped me not only made the book possible, but also inspired me deeply.

As often is the case with me, when I decide to do something, I jump right in. Writing this book was no exception. I jumped right in amid the comments from my oldest daughters: "A book, you're writing a book? Do you realize how much work that is?" My youngest just rolled her eyes and laughed. My husband, always willing to support me in all my endeavors (and I have had a lot of endeavors!), thought it was great. He has supported me though starting a school for our daughters, two businesses, and so much more. Just when our plate is so full we couldn't possibly have another moment, I find a new project I just *have* to do. And, as always, I could never do it without them.

Shortly after I started to write this book, my wrists and fingers became stiff and painful. I could plug away and get some writing done, but the days of nonstop typing were gone. The words, "Do you realize how much work that is?" never seemed more appropriate. The book turned out to fill some of my days during the last summer before my eldest daughter left for college, and it gave us the opportunity to work side-by-side as a team. Amid her harsh "I told you so's" was a level of support and dedication that made this book happen. I would sometimes have to dictate when my hands could no longer type, and she would do the typing. I found I could not always talk the way I could write, so I would dictate, and she would painfully read every line back until what she had written was what I wanted to say. At times when she would read back the passages she would construct I was in awe of how beautiful she could make my thoughts sound. After years of correcting, editing, and helping her with papers, the tides had turned; she had now surpassed me.

Both of my daughters ended up putting many hours into a project they did not ask for. They became my research assistants and set up shop in countless stores, plowing through labels and painstakingly writing down every ingredient for me. Their willingness, support, and devotion were not all that inspired me. It was also their willingness to be open and change. It was their desire to see a better future than we have shown their generation and their willingness to work for it. It was important for me to write this book not only to educate but also to inspire. I wanted to show that there is a different way we can look at and solve problems. I look at my daughters and see the future in their eyes. I see the mess we have left them with and the solutions and hope they will need to solve these problems. Sometimes, I see a generation of really amazing humans who, despite their capabilities, are becoming cynical and feeling less empowered. However, it is the small, successful changes that do occur, the small messages of hope and the ways in which they continue to strive for positive change that inspire us all to keep going. It is the stories of beating incredible odds that makes us believe that as humans we can continually do so. We need to stop the gloom-and-doom messages and replace them with ways in which change can and does occur. We may be creating a legacy of destroying our planet, using our nonrenewable resources and creating countless other problems, but we can also leave a legacy of the change we have made to correct this, and we can leave hope. When I look at my girls, I see all our children, and I am excited to have them have the world in their hands. We need to make sure they know they can change it for the better. I have witnessed both of my girls go into apathy when all the woes of the world seem too much, but I have also seen them come out willing to work, fight, and commit to making change happen.

Inspiration comes from many places. I was shocked by the graciousness and wisdom of these four women: Keisha Whitaker, Kyra Sedgwick, Marcia Gay Harden, and Didiayer Snyder. Not only did they share their views on beauty and green living, but also their heartfelt words are an inspiration to us all. They are looking at the future and making choices and changes now.

In order to write this book I needed the support of my staff at Sumbody. Over the years we have had employees come and go, and they have all made an impact on how we think and what we do. When you spend so much of your time at work, those people around you become an important part of who you are. We learn so much from each other in the workplace, from patience and understanding to compassion and acceptance. I would like to thank everyone who has come through Sumbody for the lessons they have taught me.

When writing this book I wanted a Foreword that was from someone that I not only admire and who inspires me, but that others are inspired by as well. Someone who also sees a bright future and is working toward making that happen as well. Only one name came to mind, Frank Lipman. It had been a while since we last spoke. Nervously, tentatively, and with trepidation I asked; with warmth, love, and no hesitation he accepted. Frank is truly a man I feel blessed to share this planet with.

Noelle Robbins made this book happen. During an interview she said, "You should write a book." I told her I had, but I didn't know what to do with it. She did. She introduced me to my publisher. I am forever grateful.

She introduced me to Kiran S. Rana at Hunter House. From our first meeting, I felt like he believed in both my book and me. He helped me shape my ideas into a book he could market and was always enthusiastic and supportive of the content. I am thankful he had the vision to publish my book.

I was completely green (no pun intended). Barbara Moulton at Hunter House was a blessing and a joy to work with; thank you for you kind words, support, and understanding.

Alex Mummery had the enormous job of taking all the editorial comments, my rebuttals, and everything in between into consideration and making sure the "finished" manuscript is a readable book. All the while, she was trying to maintain my happiness and approval, as well as those of the publisher, editors, and herself. She was thoughtful, patient, detail-oriented, and creative. Hers was not an easy job, yet she made it seem so and never lost her pleasant nature.

It truly takes a team, and one important member has been Kristin Giese. She has believed in Sumbody and my vision from the start. Kristin is another person who inspired me while writing this book, as she is one of the people who is living by her own rules and making changes now to positively affect our future.

I would like to thank Sam Stafford, who always partakes in all of our family's crazy endeavors, for happily putting in hours of work and support by helping with the tedious details. I would also like to thank both of my parents for making it possible for me to believe I can do anything and for being such great and supportive grandparents.

There are so many people to thank I could not possibly mention everyone who has inspired and supported me. My family and friends have provided an endless amount of support. I frequently travel to Los Angeles for work and have been fortunate to stay with my cousin Carol, who has generously opened her heart and home to not only me, but also to anyone I happen to be traveling with. It is not only her amazing hospitality that inspires me; it is her wisdom and grace. Her mind is forever open, her home filled with inspirational people from around the world, and her heart expanded to full capacity. She is a treasure, and I am in awe of her beauty.

One of my many lectures to my daughters has always been: "I do not see problems, I see solutions; look for the solutions, do not focus on the problems." For everyone who is on a path of health, change, and positive solutions, I thank you for seeing our world the way it can and will be.

Live well,
Deborah

About the Celebrity "Green Spotlights" in this Book

Throughout the book I have included interviews with women I have come to admire, Marcia Gay Harden, Kyra Sedgwick, Didiayer Snyder, and Keisha Whitaker.

When I was thinking about beauty and skincare, being natural and green, and caring about the planet's health as well as that of the people, I wanted to reach out to iconic leaders in the field...people we look to as images of beauty. The women I chose stuck out to me for different reasons, but they all shared a common interest in helping others. What could be more beautiful?

I wanted to include voices that would help me put the concepts of change and natural skin care into action. I wanted to hear from women who are already making some of these choices, already using healthy alternatives. I wanted to look at the lives of women we expect to be beautiful, women who work in a business where being beautiful on the outside is paramount and the pressure to look good is undeniable. Hearing their stories, seeing their commitment, and appreciating their beauty, lets us know we all can make positive changes. We all can make a difference and still be beautiful.

It was a look into the insides of these beautiful people that I wanted to show, since beauty truly is more than skin deep. It was this look that I wanted women to be able identify with, not the false images they are being sold. When I think of beauty, all four of these women embody my conception of it. Of course it is a bonus that they are gorgeous on the outside, but more importantly, they all care about their health over beauty, the health of the planet over ego, and are willing to share these views in an effort to create change for others' health and that of the planet. They care, and they are willing to take on causes, from charity work to reaching out to women to make a difference, working quietly and without fanfare on others' behalves. I applaud them for using their voices to help the planet be a better place for us all.

Kyra Sedgwick

I admired Kyra before I met her, in part because we have a mutual friend who is a holistic doctor and is very involved in charity work. Her dedication to charity and improving the lives of others, as well as living a holistic lifestyle, sparked my curiosity to hear her perspective on beauty and beauty products. I was not disappointed when I met her—she is one of the most gracious, warm, sincere, and truly concerned people I have met. Not only was she concerned, but extremely educated and conscientious about the importance of being as green as you can be for your own health, the planet's health, and the health of future generations.

It is always an incredible inspiration for me when I am lucky enough to come into contact with people who have the capacity to balance an extremely hectic lifestyle (if hers could even be coined so lightly!) with the drive to make a difference for our planet. She juggles being a mom (I have had the pleasure of watching her with her daughter—she is loving, kind, and patient, and always makes time for her children), a wife, and a star on a hit television series (just to name of few of her daily activities), and in the midst of all this, she is able to maintain her focus: a green commitment to herself, her family, and future generations. Kyra is right on rhythm; she is truly a rare and remarkable person.

Marcia Gay Harden

Marcia Gay Harden was the first person I asked to partake in my book. I assumed that no celebrity would be willing to lend their name and take time out of their busy schedule to help.

I decided to ask Marcia, because of all the celebrities I have met and worked with over the years, she was someone whose beauty stood out to me. I met her at an event and spoke briefly to her. I could tell she was aware of and concerned about her health and the planet's health, and was living a life in line with her awareness and concern for the planet. What really struck me was that I gave her some products to try and she sent me a handwritten thank-you note. This is unusual for anyone in this day and age, but for her to remember and to take the time to thank me was so thoughtful and gracious. It was this act of kindness, indicating her admiration for my product line and awareness of all things natural, that led me to ask her if she would be interviewed for the book. To my surprise, it took less than twenty-four hours for her to say yes, and this gave me the courage to ask others.

Keisha Whitaker

Keisha has always been one of the most phenomenally beautiful people on the outside, but she also glows from the inside. Every time I'm with her I am impressed by her nature. Her personality, warmth, and generosity are evident to all. From conversations with her, I know she is concerned about the state of the planet and the overuse of chemicals and toxins—overall she is a representation of exactly what this book is about. She is educating herself about these issues and making conscious changes in her daily life. One time when I was at her home I heard her ask a friend on the phone, "Did you see *Oprah* today? Do you know how much electricity and money we are all wasting by having everything we are not using plugged in all the time?" As Keisha was explaining all she had learned about this waste to the listener on the other end of the phone, she was simultaneously unplugging all she could. "We need power strips," I heard her say. From a TV show she watched that day to action. That is Keisha—always wanting to learn, willing to change, and wasting no time. She also lives the "Hollywood" life. She is a former model, is married to an Oscar-winning star, and is always in the limelight. She lives in a city and culture that sells us our concept of what beauty is. She also represents what we consider beautiful as a culture on the outside. Yet in all this, she manages to maintain a balance between beauty and a concern for welfare over looks.

When I told Keisha about the project I was working on and asked her if she would participate, even with her crazy schedule, she said,

"Of course." Keisha is one of the most genuine, generous, and giving people I have met. Her phone is always ringing from people asking her for help, and she is always there to give it.

Didiayer Snyder

When Didiayer offered to do an interview for my book, I was extremely excited. Living in Los Angeles as an ex-model and a designer on the hit television show *Extreme Makeover Home Edition*, she was just the type of person I was looking for to inspire women.

Within five minutes of speaking with her, it was clear that the beauty she radiates on the outside is nothing compared to the beauty that shines from her heart. Didiayer not only possesses an abundance of compassion, wisdom, kindness, and hope, she is also one of the few willing to take action. She actively uses her voice to create change.

PART I

Beauty Product ABCs

*Personal beauty is a greater recommendation
than any letter of reference.*

— ARISTOTLE —

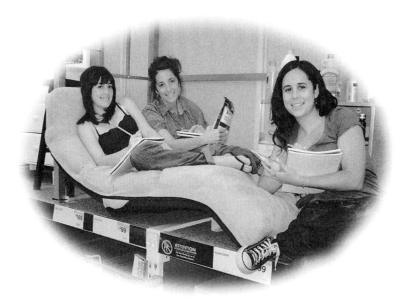

*My daughters, Autumn (right) and Mica (left) Burnes, and I set up shop at
Walmart to investigate label claims on popular beauty products*

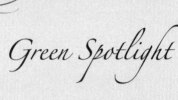

Green Spotlight

Kyra Sedgwick,
Golden Globe–Winning Actress and Activist

"Beauty is being able to walk in other peoples' shoes with compassion and understanding, and learning to tread lightly on our delicate planet. We must take care of what we do and how we do it. We take care concerning what we eat; we should also take care regarding what we put on our skin. We have to be concerned, because beauty products play a very big role in our overall health. Everything you put on your skin is a combination of chemicals—it's processed and manufactured, which has a greater negative impact on the environment as well as on your skin.

"Our culture is a culture that is enamored with youth. We glamorize looking young, and we obsess and stress out about aging. We need to embrace our aging as a culture and have mentors who are willing to age naturally. It is important for the health of our girls to reverse this culture that has a fear of change. As we age, our looks change and we perceive these aging changes as neither beautiful nor attractive. So instead of embracing aging, we slather ourselves in chemicals to stave off looking 'old.' Because of this irrational and fabricated fear of aging, we are voluntarily putting stuff on our skin that's wreaking harm on our health and the health of the planet in order to obtain this unobtainable goal of eternal youth. We're sold a bill of goods by the chemical industry that this is going to make us young and beautiful. Meanwhile, these same companies are putting gasoline into skincare products, thereby feeding the oil industry, poisoning us, and depleting the natural resources we have.

"We are depleting our resources and thus destroying the right to a healthy and prosperous life for our future generations. One of my concerns and something that I care deeply about is our children. For me it's about our children. We need to be replenishing our resources so they will have plenty. We have limited resources, and I'm terribly worried that there won't be enough clean air or water for our children. We need easy solutions, and we need them fast. So finding ways like Deborah suggests in this book, like swapping products we're already using for better alternatives, whether it be in skin care, food, light bulbs, transportation, or any other facet of life, is of the utmost importance. These alternatives are easy and have a far-reaching impact on our own health and well-being and that of the planet. These are the type of simple choices that we can make to ensure that our children have clean air and clean water.

"These are simple choices we can all make without any creating negative impact on our personal lives; these simple changes benefit us all.

"In this way, we can all be beautiful. We can all walk in each other's shoes with compassion and understanding. We can all participate in the ultimate vision of beauty by caring enough to protect our own health and that of our families, and at the same time by having enough compassion to care for the planet and to preserve life and resources for our future generations. That is beautiful."

Chapter 1

From Cleopatra to Clearasil

The Innate Desire to Beautify

There is nothing that makes its way
more directly to the soul
than beauty.

— JOSEPH ADDISON

The concept of using materials to enhance one's perceived beauty is not new. The styles and standards for beauty have changed, but the ritual of attempting to perfect oneself remains an enduring facet of cultural life. We have evidence dating back to 10,000 BCE that shows Egyptian use of kohl as both an eye shadow and eyeliner. Centuries later, but still relatively early in recorded history, Romans were bathing in scented water and anointing themselves with sweet-smelling oils. The word *cosmetic* is related to the word *cosmetae*, which refers to the Roman slaves responsible for bathing men and women in perfume. That humans have long experienced a drive toward physical perfection is undisputed; uncovering the impetus behind that drive, however, has led to differing theories.

We cannot travel back in time and ask for a simple explanation of why people started painting their faces, but one of the more plausible theories is that both men and women used kohl as eyeliner in harsh desert areas to protect their eyes from the glare—just as football players darken their lower eye areas today. This usage quickly evolved from practicality to vanity and gave way to an array of colors, powders, and creams aimed at perfecting one's appearance.

Modern technology has enhanced our capacity to finely tune parts of our bodies in an effort to conform to today's standards of beauty. We can reshape our noses, enhance our breasts, and remove unwanted fat tissue from our bodies. We have progressed from using kohl as sun protection, to using colored eyeliners and hair dyes, to even surgically altering our bodies. This creates a whole new slew of problems involving the effects of permanently altering our bodies.

From this craving to beautify sprung the beauty industry we have today. Beauty products are an integral part of our society. While history shows that it is unrealistic to expect to eliminate cosmetics, we can learn to make informed choices that drastically lessen the adverse effects of cosmetics.

Beauty: A Historical Perspective

A woman without paint is like food without salt.

— Plautus, Roman playwright (254–184 BCE)

The human desire to enhance one's beauty dates back to the first organized civilization—the Sumerians—which manufactured soap. While our expertise in manufacturing and using makeup has improved greatly over the years, the areas where we apply makeup have changed very little. Take, for example, the stereotypical painting of an Egyptian woman. Now contrast that with the stereotypical American woman in the 1950s. Both are wearing dark eyeliner. The '50s woman has added blue eye shadow above the liner. While her makeup is slightly more advanced, the basic principles remain the same. Below is a description of a few of the cultures that have had a large impact on shaping the face of the beauty industry.

Ancient Egypt

In ancient Egypt, people used henna in their hair and on their cheeks, lips, and nails, and they used kohl, which is comprised of lead, copper, burned almonds, and other ingredients on their eyes and eyebrows. In addition to applying colors, Egyptian aspirations toward beauty encompassed the desire for softer, smoother, younger-looking skin. To this end, they used oils for moisturizing, applied body scents, and took soothing moisturizing baths. Cleopatra was the queen of the milk bath, which used crushed rose petals. Modern-day women are still searching for the same effects. While the Egyptians created their own organic products, we run to the store for the new "miracle in a jar."

Ancient Greece

While the Greeks incorporated many Egyptian techniques into their beauty regime, they brought to the endeavor a slightly different purpose. Whereas the Egyptians strived for beauty in order to impress one another and the gods, the Greeks were only trying to impress one another. This is one of their major contributions to the evolution of the beauty industry. The raw ingredients varied, but the type of product remained the same. Their major contribution to the evolution of the beauty industry is in their focus on looking beautiful for each other. The other main component of the modern beauty industry that we find in Greek culture is the importance of packaging, as they packaged many products in fancy bottles and jars. These two components make up the basis for our attraction to beauty products today.

Europe

From the Middle Ages to the Industrial Revolution, pale skin was a sign of status in European culture. Because the skin of the working class was tanned from outside labor, pale skin became a coveted symbol of the aristocracy. Men and women both applied white face powders in an effort to be perceived as a member of the highest class. Just as it is today, makeup was used to alter the way a person is perceived in society. While our standards for beauty have left pale faces in the dust, we still alter our appearance to attract a certain attention and create a certain impression. If a woman is going to a job interview, she will do her makeup differently than if she were going to a rock concert. In our cultural perception of beauty, we think of someone differently depending on how she makes herself up.

Beauty After the Nineteenth Century

The process of promoting and selling cosmetics geared up around the turn of the century. People began formulating more complex products and opening salons. Many brand names that we still recognize originated in this era. Helena Rubenstein opened her first salon in New York in 1915. Just before that, in 1912, Elizabeth Arden traveled from New York to France, where she learned beauty techniques and facial massage in the Parisian salons. She returned with a collection of rouges and tinted powders that she had created. At the time, it was only acceptable for stage performers to wear makeup; Arden changed this viewpoint, and she also created the concept of the beauty makeover. She later teamed up with a chemist named A. Fabian Swanson to create a "fluffy" face cream.

In Europe and America in the 1920s, tanned skin became popular. Industry hopped on this new attitude and created a new line of products to mimic natural suntans. This began with lotions and oils, and moved into tanning spray and eventually tanning booths and high-powered lights in the 1970s.

Glamour was ushered in during the 1950s. Max Factor, who coined the term *makeup*, based on the verb *to make up*, began his career developing colors and styles for a Russian ballet company. He transferred his skills to Hollywood movie stars and opened the first Max Factor salon near Hollywood Boulevard. Most important, he brought glamour to the makeup scene. Flashy and dramatic, Max Factor made regular people crave the looks of the stars. Thus began one of the most overwhelming trends in the beauty industry—Americans don't have a true aristocracy, but it was replaced by the influence of the Hollywood culture, and people tried hard to be perceived as part of this culture.

This infatuation with movie stars is even stronger today, and it is reflected in cosmetic producers' desire to court the celebrities. One day a representative from a major fashion magazine called my office to ask about a sugar scrub she was in love with. The first thing she asked was which celebrities used it. When I answered (fortunately there were some!), she replied that they were not popular enough—she told me to call back when we had an A-lister.

I understand the attitudes of the consumer, cosmetic producer, and magazine editor. A consumer is looking for an escape—a way to experience the perceived glamour of Nicole Kidman's life with one swipe of lipstick. The producer is looking for a hook—a way to make its product stand out—and one way to achieve this is by having strong celebrity support. The magazine is looking to sell issues, by showing people what they want to see—what their favorite celebrities are wearing and using, and where to find these products. The ripple effect of these desires shapes our beauty industry today. Manufacturers will spend more money courting, or in some cases hiring, celebrities than they do on the development of their product's ingredients. This adds a whole new element to the industry. Sales are driven not only by what's in the bottle, but by who's using it.

From Self-Made to Mass-Produced

When people first began altering their appearances by using makeup, they applied ingredients they found in their everyday lives. The ingredients for kohl, such as lead, were easily obtained. People had all the means to make their own beauty products from ingredients that were readily available to them. I grew up on the East Coast, and when I was little we used to play with rocks we called Indian paint pots. We spit in the center, swirled the spit around the rock with our finger, and painted it on our faces. The natural color from this stone produced a beautiful blush, lip color, or eye shadow. Perhaps people who lived in the same area two hundred years earlier had used this stone to paint their faces. So if we have the capacity to create our own natural products, what has happened?

Just as some chefs have a more precise palate and are more renowned for their skills than others, some people have a better sense of smell and perception of color. When people realized they could make a living formulating better scents and colors, they did so. Naturally, everyone wanted these superior products. Thus the beauty industry shifted from self-made to mass-produced. And of course, there was the convenience factor. It is much easier to buy a product than to make it from scratch. Nowadays our lives are busier than ever, and we no longer have the time to make our own products. The evolution of the beauty industry is not unlike that of many other industries. People saw a window of opportunity to make money and seized it. Similar shifts occurred in the clothing and food industries. We no longer have time to sew our own clothes and cook all of our food from scratch. As the demand and competition for these products grows, so does the variety of products available on the market.

In today's multibillion-dollar beauty industry, we have eyeliner, mascara, foundation, cleaning pads, cleansers, lotions, face creams, body lotions, body creams, lipstick, lip plumping gels, antiwrinkle masks, lip gloss, etcetera. The vast array of products and the number of companies producing them underscore the importance of this industry to our society. We can buy products from massive companies like Max Factor, Elizabeth Arden, and Unilever, or from small mom-and-pop outfits that make "miracle" emu-oil lip balms. Do you know how many cosmetic companies there are? The number is overwhelming and is a testament to the amount of money spent on cosmetics each year. While I was growing up, I remember hearing that during the Great Depression, when industry was at a standstill, there were three things that still sold: tobacco, alcohol, and Woolworth's red lipstick. It appears that no matter what, women will buy their red lipstick.

At Risk

From the inception of the beauty industry, there have been harmful ingredients in products. There were heavy metals in the kohl used in Egyptian eyeliner and in the face powders that Europeans used. The difference is that people were unaware of the potentially harmful effects of their makeup. Now we know of these dangers, but we continue to use the same products. While we have removed lead and iron, we have not eliminated the threat cosmetics pose to us. We have more raw ingredients available to us than ever before, as well as an enormous capacity to manufacture synthetic ingredients. The sheer numbers of chemicals and other harmful ingredients used in the industry is overwhelming, and this alone poses more of a threat than ever before.

All the toxins in the beauty products of centuries ago were found in nature. Now we have manufactured thousands of toxins, and the creation of synthetic ingredients threatens not only our health but our environment. Industrial chemical plants devoted solely to manufacturing ingredients for cosmetics cause runoff, waste, and pollution that do untold damage. There are so many possible combinations of these chemicals—each one with its own potentially adverse health and environmental effects—that we do not even know the full scope of this problem.

Environmental pollution effects everyone, whether or not he or she wears makeup or uses body-care products. This has become a global problem, and it needs a comprehensive solution.

Chapter 2

What's in a Name?

*Unmasking Label and
Ingredient Claims and
Understanding What
Natural Means*

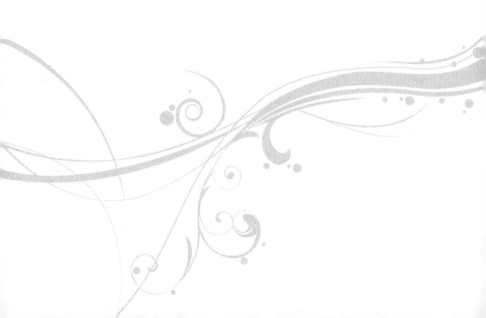

"Have you tried that?" inquired a voice from behind me as I returned a bottle of Dr. Bronner's Pure Liquid Castile Soap to the shelf. I was in the middle of my research for the "Good," "Better," "Best" lists provided in Chapters 11 through 15, which are a compilation of products that I have researched and rated from a range of good alternatives to the best alternatives for consumers to choose from. Pausing, I answered the woman's question, "Yes, I have." We were not in a store selling wheat grass and organic vegetables, and this woman did not have dandelions in her hair and three layers of flowing skirts. She was a plainly dressed and tastefully made-up middle-aged woman.

Our conversation in the aisle lasted for nearly a half hour as she picked my brain about the healthiest choice for everything on her list. She pulled out a scrap of paper listing ten ingredients that she was trying to avoid. By searching the Internet, she had learned that a certain brand did not use sodium lauryl sulfate (her cart was filled with products from this brand). However, dissecting her shopping cart and critically reading the labels taught me otherwise. The second ingredient after water in one of these supposed sodium lauryl sulfate-free products was sodium lauryl sulfate. Shocked, she asked how this could be legal. Most likely, the ad she saw touted one product of this brand as being free of this chemical. The marketing scheme worked—by making one product without sodium lauryl sulfate, the company had convinced a consumer to trust the entire brand. A similar problem occurred as she searched for makeup for her daughters. From the same company, one product would advertise "no parabens" but contain talc, while another would claim "no talc" but contain parabens—both were on her list of ingredients to avoid. Beyond her own desire to avoid these chemicals, she was also a mother looking for safe products for her children. Her enthusiasm and curiosity showed me the breadth of the audience this book would have; so many people are searching for ways to be healthy, but the necessary information is not out there in a simple, concise, and accessible form.

From makeup, we moved on to cleaning products; the ones she had chosen were plastered with amazing claims but did not list ingredients. After looking at the bottle in her shopping cart, I could tell her the product was safer than your average cleaning product, but I could not guarantee that each ingredient was safe. In this case, I told her, it fit into the "85 percent clean, 15 percent junk" philosophy that guides my basic lifestyle. I am not an extremist who thinks we should all sew our own clothes and eat only what we grow ourselves. I believe in affecting change through moderation, and I want consumers to have accessible, healthy choices everywhere from the local drugstore to Nordstrom. I try to be 85 percent healthy and reserve 15 percent for some vitamin J—junk. When my kids were young, I tended to sway toward the extremist side of things—no sugar, preservatives, or soda—even juice was mostly forbidden. I developed my 85 percent/15 percent philosophy one day in the car when my kids were around ages five and eight. I overheard them saying that as soon as they moved out of the house they were going to buy ice cream and a giant bag of Doritos and sit around and watch TV all day long. This was when I realized the importance of moderation. To their disbelief, on the way home we stopped at the store and I bought them ice cream and Doritos, and when we got home I let them watch TV.

For some people, junk may consist of dyeing their hair or eating fast food. Eighty-five percent may be too high or too low for your comfort zone. All I am advocating is that you find your own comfort zone and try to stick to it. The woman at the store had her zone and was working to stay within its boundaries. If everyone commits to some type of change, together we can make a difference. The problem is that even with her comfort zone in mind and good intentions, the woman was still unable to find products that fit her expectations—even when she thought they did.

This is where I come in. This book is not only for those committed to having zero chemical exposure but also for those striving to decrease their chemical load. You don't have to be a diehard to want to make informed choices. My goal is to help every individual find a healthy alternative that truly meets her expectations.

Daily Exposure

Each day, the average American uses eight personal-care products, such as toothpaste, skin cream, shampoo, lip balm, deodorant, cologne, sunscreen, and soap. On average, these products contain a total of 138 different ingredients that enter your body. Of these, most are toxic. The truth is that no one really knows what effect mixing this many different toxins in and on your body will have, or whether a "cocktail effect" will increase the impact of these toxins. Yet we continue to add new "miracle" ingredients to products and add new products to our daily regimens. I find myself wondering whether we would overlook these chemicals' caustic effects if they did not promise to make us look younger and more beautiful. Consider propylene glycol, which studies suggest causes damage to the kidneys, lungs, heart, and nervous system. If I gathered up every drop of propylene glycol you were exposed to via body products in one month and put it in a shot glass with a warning label, would you drink it? Most of us wouldn't order propylene glycol at a bar even if it tasted like apple cider. For some reason, poison on our skin does not set off the same internal alarm bells as poison in our mouths. When making personal-care choices, here's a good rule of thumb: We should not apply anything to our skin that we would not feel comfortable ingesting.

Why You Should Care about What's in Your Cosmetics

Although we have not yet as a culture embraced, nor do we fully understand, the connection between our personal health and what we put on our body, the fact remains that it has a profound effect. Understanding the impact is imperative to maintaining a healthy lifestyle.

In evaluating the health and safety of what we are "wearing" on our skin, it would be an oversight to not look at the impact these products are having on the health of our children and the planet. Children are more vulnerable to toxins, so we need to be aware and limit their exposure. Additionally, our planet is becoming a toxic dumping ground for the excessive amounts of chemicals we are using. By slathering ourselves daily with everything from body lotions to face creams that are loaded with chemicals, we are, in turn, slathering them on our planet as well.

Your Overall Health

The ingredients in nicotine and birth-control patches function by penetrating your skin and traveling into your bloodstream. So while there's controversy over how much of the chemicals in your skin-care products are actually penetrating your skin, keep in mind that there is scientific evidence for effective medication reaching the bloodstream through skin. The controversy springs from the fact that some molecules are too large to be absorbed by your sebaceous glands, also known as your pores. Many who advocate chemical products will argue that nothing in them penetrates your skin, while many who support all-natural products will claim that everything gets past your skin's barrier. The truth is that no matter how you look at it, most of what you apply to your skin is likely getting through. While some molecules may be too large to enter your pores, they can easily enter your bloodstream through your eyes, ears, or mouth and nose. In 1999, researchers at Stanford University found that they were able to deliver as effective of a dose of a DNA vaccine through an animal's skin as through an injection. Take a moment to consider the significance of this data. Something rubbed onto your skin can deliver an effective dose of a vaccination. It is time that we really pay attention to what we are putting on our skin. The well-documented hazards of many of the chemicals in skin-care products, coupled with the permeability of skin, means we have to reassess our comfort level with applying these chemicals topically. We can't wait for laws that prevent manufacturers from using these chemicals—we have to use our knowledge and reasoning to make decisions for ourselves. Right now the industry takes an "innocent until proven guilty" approach to using chemicals, but given the amount of chemicals leaching into our skin, we cannot afford to wait for evidence. If there is a question about an ingredient or if we do not know the research, we should be safe and avoid it.

Outside influences have too much control over our personal health. As careful as we can try to be when it comes to what we choose to put into our bodies and our children's bodies, these out-side sources have found loopholes that allow them to subject us to poisons without our knowledge. These loopholes consist of actions such as allowing ingredients that are banned from food additives to be used in body products that end up in our bloodstream just as they would if we were eating them, as well as using ingredients that are known to be harmful without providing disclosure to the consumer. As consumers, we did not sign up to be volunteers in lab experiments. Yet that's exactly what we have become. In a culture where people are protesting against animal testing and choosing to use only products that do not use animal-tested research, it seems ironic that our bodies have become the testing ground for toxic chemicals. We've been put-ting our children, our habitat, and ourselves on the line.

Your Children's Health

From the moment they appear in their mother's womb, children are bombarded with chemicals. They are exposed not only to air pollut-ants and chemicals in the environment, but also to any chemicals the mother eats or applies topically. This means lotions, oils, moisturizers, and any number of products a mother uses during her pregnancy. This includes not just what goes on her belly, but also soap, makeup, and the entire gamut of beauty-care products. According to a recent study conducted by the Environmental Working Group (EWG) in collaboration with Commonweal, "Researchers at two major labora-tories found an average of two-hundred industrial chemicals and pol-lutants in umbilical cord blood from ten babies born in August and September of 2004 in U.S. hospitals. Tests revealed a total of 287 chemi-cals in the group. The umbilical cord blood of these ten children, col-lected by the Red Cross after the cord was cut, harbored pesticides, consumer product ingredients, and wastes from burning coal, gaso-line, and garbage."

Babies' systems are extremely fragile and have a lesser capacity to process these chemicals than adults' systems. With the increase in air pollutants and other environmental strains your child must be exposed to, it becomes even more important to control what expo-sure we can. This means both before and after a child is born. Most baby products are formulated for entertainment, not necessity. While orange lather is tons of fun, is it worth exposing an already assaulted and fragile child to toxic chemicals? We have to make choices about what we need, what we can do without, and which products we can find safe alternatives for. In the PBS documentary *Trade Secrets,* Bill Moyers says, "Today, not a single child is born free of synthetic chemicals." Our goal, then, must be to prevent these levels from increasing by eliminating avoidable exposure to synthetic chemicals. Jane Hersey, director of the Feingold Association, an organization dedicated to preventing and treating learning and behavioral disorders, says, "Research now confirms what many parents and teachers have long suspected: that some children experience behavior, learning, or respiratory problems when they eat foods containing petroleum-based additives like dyes, synthetic flavorings, and certain preservatives." While there has been a move to avoid or regulate these additives in food, nothing is being done to prevent them from entering through another route—the skin.

We control what is sold to us. If we demand truly natural products, companies will be forced to manufacture them. Evidence of this can be seen in the pervasive use of the claim *natural.* Consumers are searching for natural products, so every company, from the largest manufacturer to the smallest mom-and-pop producer, markets its products as *natural.* Now, if we as consumers take our demands one step further and require that products claiming to be *natural* actually contain all-natural ingredients, the industry will be forced to comply. Companies seek out profits using two main strategies—they cut costs and aim to sell volume. Often the desire to cut costs is what leads to the use of chemicals. But if these chemicals compromise the vendor's ability to sell volume, it will have to deliver what the market is screaming for—truly *natural* products.

The Planet's Health

Determining whether a product has healthy ingredients or not does not enable one to vouch for how products are produced, what companies are owned by other companies, or how products are packaged. The same companies that make natural products may be owned by a company that has poor environmental practices or uses excessive packaging that wreaks havoc on the environment. Regardless of these

factors, eliminating or reducing chemicals in your products will ensure that fewer chemicals are released into nature. Even this small
change has the potential to make a significant impact on our environment. Exposure to personal-care toxins is a serious public-health
issue. According to the U.S. Environmental Protection Agency, fifty
thousand chemicals, the vast majority of them known to adversely affect the human body, are being diffused into our environment. *Our
children are the most at risk from exposure to these toxins.*

It is easy to become paralyzed by the seemingly overwhelming
prospect of effecting global change—we have to recycle, use compact
fluorescent lightbulbs, turn off our air-conditioning, sell our car, take
the bus, compost, carpool, change our cleaning products, buy used
clothing, use cloth napkins. We are so inundated with information
and recommendations that we stop trying at all. Some people will go
further than others in terms of reducing their impact on the environment, but most of us are not going to change our entire lifestyle. Relax and breathe; this is okay. Change can happen slowly and can come
about through small shifts—we don't have to do everything on the list
all at once. Pick a few changes that feel doable. When I look around, I
see change happening all the time. I see eighty-year-old women using
cloth napkins and reusable bags and kindergarteners caring about re-
cycling. We are in the midst of a large-scale mobilization to help combat global warming and save our environment. Many people say that
this is only one more in-vogue thing to care and think about and that
there are really more people wearing the T-shirts than caring about
the issues. Yes, it is trendy to go green, but even that speaks to our ability to create change. It is important that celebrities and major publi-
cations are discussing the environment rather than the latest scandal
or hottest vacation spots. This displays a core shift in priorities. We
have the power and the willingness to affect change—now let's get
out there and make the right choices!

Making Choices that Control Your Exposure to Chemicals

When I set out to research natural brands, I had no idea how difficult it would be. I figured, if a company's ingredients are good, it will

advertise them so that everyone can access this information. I was wrong.

One of my most eye-opening experiences occurred in 2008 when I first went online to look at Whole Foods' body-care products. The home page of the body-care section featured this quote: "At Whole Foods Market, we believe that the products you use every day for health and beauty should be as natural and as safe as the foods you eat. We encourage you to feed both the inside and the outside of your body the nutrients that it needs to function properly. We believe that using natural products is the most effective means of doing that, and by sharing the facts, you'll be inspired to be good to your whole body, every day." I was struck by this open, honest, and knowledgeable approach and excited to learn more, so I called Whole Foods to inquire about its standards for body care. The woman on the phone replied that the company had a list of ingredients that could not be used in any of the products and a more stringent list of those that could not be used in their premium-line products. Intrigued, I asked for a copy of the list, thinking Whole Foods probably used it as advertising material. I was surprised to find out that at the time this list was considered proprietary information and not released to the public. However, the woman explained, I could ask about any ingredient and she would tell me whether or not it had a spot on the list. I played the guessing game for a few rounds before tiring and thanking her for her time. The experience seemed surreal—there was a list but I could not see it, I could only guess what was on it. As a consumer I have a right to know what is in my products, and I should not have to work very hard to exercise this right.

I support Whole Foods and do not intend to discredit it in any way, and the company has since started to post all their standards and list any and all important information, including what ingredients it does not allow in any of its products as well as what is not allowed in its premium-brand products. What a major step for the consumer. What a wonderful role model Whole Foods is providing to the industry. What a turnaround in a short time from my first encounter with Whole Foods. My point, however, is that more often than not, such as during my first experience with Whole Foods, ingredients and standards were not readily available to the consumer. Additionally, I have found some of my favorite products at Whole Foods are no better than the standard version you find at your local drugstore. Unfortunately, you wouldn't know this from its advertising. Whole Foods has created a brand name that people automatically associate with natural, healthy, largely organic foods, and this ethos carries over into its body line as well. People let their guard down when they're shopping for body products at Whole Foods because they assume that everything is safe and healthy. This made it even more important for Whole Foods to post its standards. It was the only large store I found at the time I was researching that even had a list of standards—it should have been proud of them.

I understand that the list may be constantly changing in accordance with new research, but this should not prevent any company from posting one. Whole Foods stores post new signs in their delis each day. Additionally, this should be an advertising bonus because people will know that Whole Foods is watching out for its customers and keeping pace with the latest research. Customers can see the standards and decide whether they are comfortable with those standards and will purchase anything off the shelf, whether they prefer the premium line, or whether their personal standards are even higher and they still need to read the ingredients. Although Whole Foods has an impressive amount of information and its ingredient lists are now available online, I would like to see this information provided at a spot where the consumers are making their choices—in the store. By not making all the pertinent information accessible, it forces consumers to either rely on the name brand alone or dissect every label.

I used to work in the wine industry, where Robert Parker, a leading authority on wine, gives ratings that are highly sought after. A cartoon I once saw depicted a person tasting wine and spitting it out in disgust. Another person said, "Robert Parker gave that a 99," to which the first person replied, "I'll take five cases." When people used to ask me how Parker rated a certain wine, I would explain that if they liked his palate they should trust his ratings, but their palates might not be the same, and they should choose a wine based on what *they* like. Whole Foods is the same—it has a cachet that leads some people to believe that everything Whole Foods likes must be great, but this doesn't take into account that we each have our own palate, whether for food or body care.

Instead of relying on the rating alone, people should be privy to the standards behind that rating. Whole Foods is not the only company that masks itself behind its reputation. I have found websites for body-care products that show a list of ingredients that look wonderful, followed by a miniscule asterisk that says, "Click here for a full list of ingredients." Consumers should not have to jump through hoops to get information as simple as what is in a product. Other websites simply leave certain ingredients out of their lists. I was looking at the ingredient list for a deodorant when I realized that the only ingredients listed were oils and powders, yet it was a solid-consistency product in a twist-up stick. How were these ingredients staying together in hard-bar form? I called the company to inquire and found that—oops!—it had left out the main ingredient: beeswax. Beeswax is not even a harmful ingredient. In this case I cannot figure out why the company would even leave it off the label. The only reason I can think of is because beeswax is not in itself effective as a deodorizing ingredient.

Another trick companies use is to list an ingredient in type so large that it nearly stretches across the entire bottle. When the first three-and-a-half inches of ingredients look great, we get lazy—which is just what the manufacturer is hoping will happen. The problem is, most products consist of at least 85 percent water. A company might put five drops of twenty different extracts into the water and list them all high on the label, right after water, because technically they're in 85 percent of the product, and you have to wade through these useless ingredients before getting to the actual substance. Often people give up after seeing fifteen healthy-looking extracts listed and trust that the entire product is safe, but that's usually not the case. Parabens, sodium lauryl sulfate, PEGs, fragrance (note that for labeling purposes, it is common practice for companies to use "fragrance" to refer to synthetic scents and "essential oils" or "natural scent blends" to refer to natural ones), and more all lurk in the last two lines of ingredient lists, so don't fall prey to this technique. If you're in a rush or you really don't want to wade through the entire list, read from the bottom up to assure that you aren't missing the dangerous chemicals.

I am not saying that every ingredient must be pure and natural, but rather that there should be complete honesty on a product's label and advertising. There are times when chemicals are harmless or do less harm than good. For instance, I started out making all my products fragrance-free (free of synthetic scents). The problem was that customers would come in daily asking for vanilla-scented products or cucumber essential oil—all the scents they were accustomed to buying and believed were natural. I explained that while vanilla extract exists, it is extremely expensive and does not smell as strong as a synthetic alternative, so virtually no companies use it alone to scent products. Cucumber essential oil simply does not exist; the scents these customers were referring to were all fragrances, and because I didn't have them, they went to a store that did. I thought about this for a while and decided that although fragrance is harmful, it would be better for these customers to buy a natural product with a small amount of fragrance than to purchase the synthetic products they would otherwise use. This logic led me to start formulating some scents with small amounts of fragrance. These products are more natural and effective than 99 percent of the products out there, and even now a large majority of my products are fragrance-free. My customers can pick products according to their comfort level. Additionally, the reason why some of my products contain fragrances is freely available to all customers. The depth of thought and care we invest in our products at Sumbody gives the consumer ultimate choice and control over their products and body—don't settle for a company that does less.

The Skinny on Skin Works

I touched on skin earlier while discussing the effectiveness of patches and vaccination through skin, but I want to take a moment here to really look at skin and its importance in your body. Whether producing goose bumps or sweat, our skin reacts to everything around us. It is our largest body organ, and it is the only one that has the difficult task of interacting with the outside world. As such, it is designed to protect us from environmental threats such as extreme temperature. It insulates our body and keeps us safe from dirt, bugs, and diseases.

It collects vitamin D and literally keeps us all in one piece. Unfortunately, our skin doesn't look like an organ, so it is hard for us to give it the care and respect we give to our inner organs. If we were suffering from kidney failure or liver deterioration, we would start eating more healthily, exercising, taking medication, and looking for a transplant. We would not pour chemicals onto our liver with the abandon with which we apply them to our skin. And yet in many ways, skin is the most vital organ—we cannot get a skin transplant, nor can we survive without skin. Lucky for us, skin is pretty durable, but there's not much that repeated exposure to caustic chemicals won't wear down, and the effects of weakened skin are drastic.

Who's in Control?

While researching this book, I was astounded to learn about the regulation discrepancies between one industry and the next. For example, a certain chemical can be outlawed for food- and worker-safety purposes but may be allowed in cosmetics. Chemicals that are banned from industrial manufacturing can be used in body-care products. For example, in 1992 the FDA banned the use of propylene glycol in louse-killing products, because it was not shown to be safe or effective. Yet it is still permitted for use in personal-care products at a concentration level of up to 50 percent. So it is banned for use in killing lice but approved to apply to skin and hair, as well as in creams, lotions, shampoos, and toothpaste. While the food and industrial sectors are highly regulated, the cosmetic industry lacks adequate regulation to the point that the status quo involves virtually no regulation. And these choices are being made not with the consumer's health in mind but with an eye toward the largest profit margin. Thus, especially in the body-care industry, consumers are being subjected to chemicals that are labeled as unsafe in other industries. Sherry Rogers, MD, states that in order to produce cancer or Parkinson's disease in a rat, you must inject it with certain chemicals. This is not news. The astonishing part is that these are some of the very same chemicals you will find in some of the skin-care products that are labeled organic.

Absorbed into the body, these chemicals can be stored in fatty tissue or organs such as the liver, kidneys, reproductive organs, and brain. Cosmetic companies complain of unfounded concerns, but scientists are finding harmful ingredients like phthalates in urine, preservatives known as parabens in breast-tumor tissue, and anti-bacterials such as triclosan and fragrance chemicals in human breast milk. Additional research has shown that detergents in shampoos can cause eye damage, fragrances are triggering asthma attacks, and hair-dye chemicals can cause bladder cancer and lymphoma. If nothing else, the prevalence of these chemicals proves that they are penetrating our skin and affecting our bodies. If these problems had been shown in pharmaceuticals, they would be taken off the market and money would be spent on safety studies. But because the cosmetic industry is largely self-governing and because we all want to believe in the dreams of younger-looking skin and shiny hair, products containing harmful substances remain on the market. With more and more research about the toxic effects becoming available, it appears that we have been unknowingly killing ourselves for beauty.

When faced with the evidence that a certain ingredient is harmful, cosmetic companies often scoff and claim that it would take an entire swimming pool of x hazardous chemical to harm you. While this sounds encouraging, studies that show phthalates and parabens cropping up in urine and tumors, respectively, beg to differ. We are often told that the amount of an ingredient contained in a particular product is too small to be harmful, but what about when we use several products daily that contain the same ingredient. This illustrates the extent to which these toxins are penetrating our bodies, potentially causing harm. We as consumers have to realize that there's no one looking out for us but us. We must take our safety into our own hands and protect ourselves.

One question that I have set out to try to answer is that of a definition for the word *natural*, and its significance. At first it seemed clear—anything from nature is natural. But a homemade cake is natural, and yet you'll never see one on your walk to the grocery store. So then anything made of ingredients found in nature and then exposed to heat to form a new substance should be natural. But what if you cause a reaction between a natural product and an acid? What if you are isolating molecules found in nature to create a new substance? Each example begs a few more questions until we are drawing lines between molecules. It just isn't practical to have to carry around a handbook filled with flow charts and what-ifs to determine whether or not something is natural.

Right when my head was about to explode from pondering all these potential problems, I stumbled upon the Environmental Working Group's Skin Deep website. Rather than dissecting the particulars of *natural*, Skin Deep rates each ingredient in terms of consumer safety, using a scale from zero to ten, with zero being harmless and ten being deadly. My favorite aspect of Skin Deep is that it is not alarmist—many of the ingredients it rates as moderately or mildly hazardous, I would rate much higher. There are some ingredients that are synthetically produced and yet have a safety rating of zero. Skin Deep doesn't simply cobble together a bunch of data. You can read the criteria for its ratings and find the studies and resources to substantiate every claim. Despite this site's solid reputation, don't trust everything you read on it—always be sure to look up its sources if you want a complete picture. While I applaud Skin Deep's effort to launch a site like this and can see the amount of work that went into it, they have a way to go in providing consistent, accurate information. In writing this book, I came across numerous alarming charts and impressive stats on how bad these chemicals are on various websites claiming that the Centers for Disease Control (CDC) said this or the Food and Drug Administration (FDA) did that, but I was unable to find the research myself. I called the organizations and searched the Web but still could not find a primary source for these claims, so I could not include these alarming stats and lists. The importance of verifiable information from credible sources cannot be overestimated. Throw definitions out the window, and take a look at various sites to determine whether or not an ingredient poses a threat to your body and health—just be sure to fact-check.

As a consumer, mother, and the owner of a body-care products business, I have a definition of *natural* that is more stringent. When faced with a choice between natural shea butter and safe synthetic butter that achieves the same results, I will always choose the shea butter, assuming it comes from a sustainable source. I believe it is always better to use something that comes from nature. Skin Deep also rates products as well as ingredients, and while again its intention seems good, its rating system appears to not be fully developed. A product can contain an ingredient that is rated at eight and yet receive an overall rating of three. I have called for criteria for the product ratings but have been unable to get a satisfying answer. Additionally, some of the cleanest products I found were rated poorly on Skin Deep. I was on the website of a company called Suki because I am listing its products in my "Best" section, and on it I stumbled upon an article that criticizes Skin Deep. I have no connection to Suki and no motivation to promote it aside from the fact that it is one of the cleanest companies I found. Skin Deep accused Suki of using carcinogenic ingredients. One of Suki's complaints is that Skin Deep is not always an accurate watchdog because it rates products based on the ingredients companies submit to them without checking for omitted ingredients. If you are basing your product decision on a Skin Deep rating, be sure to cross-check the ingredients reported by Skin Deep with the ingredients on the bottle. In reading the Skin Deep website, I have found ingredients rated as a one that enhance penetration and have been known to cause cancer. I have not received a satisfactory answer as to why these ingredients are rated a one. However, the website contains all of the research showing the adverse effects of the ingredients. I would suggest that if you are using Skin Deep as a guidepost, try to read as many of the studies that go along with each ingredient, as opposed to blindly trusting its ratings.

The odds might seem stacked against us, but there is a lot we can do to effect positive change—even against a sixty-billion-dollar industry. For one thing, the beauty industry doesn't think of you as one powerless person—it thinks of you as money. When we, as consumers, wise up to this fact, it becomes apparent that we have all the power. As the demand for *real* all-natural products increases, so does the availability of the natural raw ingredients needed to produce natural products. If there is money to be made, chemical companies will rush to get a natural alternative to the market. If consumers change their habits, they will also reduce the profitability of products containing harmful chemicals, which will reduce their command of the market share. This powerful "natural reaction" will profoundly affect both our own health and that of the planet in a positive way.

Ten Simple Beauty-Product Rules to Live By

Trying to figure out what is not harmful to us can become confusing and overwhelming, with the result that we as consumers tend to shut down. We can be so flooded with information that we feel we can't control or even make rules to live by. But don't forget the 85 percent clean/15 percent junk rule; you don't have to be perfect. You can start to make small changes in your daily routine to reduce your exposure to harmful ingredients, and some of these changes can be as simple as deciding where you reach on the store shelf.

1. **Use less to limit your exposure.** Go through your bathroom and be honest with yourself about what you really need. Separate all your products into two categories, the "Must have" and the "Why?" I am always shocked by the number of extra products most of us have. It is refreshing to see the response from people when they make their two piles, the "Must haves" and the "Can eliminate." It is even more rewarding when I come back for their first "checkup" consultation and we reevaluate those piles. Inevitably, the "Can eliminate" pile has gotten larger. I have seen people with as many as ten different leave-in conditioners, as well as shine enhancers, defrizzers, and smoothing creams that they were applying after each wash. One of my favorite examples is a woman who was putting on six different "miracle" creams to combat aging throughout the course of the day. When I began helping her evaluate her products, the thought of giving up those products was enough to send her to her therapist's chair. After a lot of coaxing and reassuring that she and the planet would be healthier, I promised that if she gave it two months, she would see that her chemical-filled "miracles in a jar" were actually making her skin age faster. I promised her she could save money, time, energy, and her ego, and reduce her impact on the planet, all at once.

The fun was in the two-month checkup when she greeted me with a smile and said she had never gotten so may comments on how wonderful she looked. With the money she'd saved, she managed to purchase some new clothes to go with what she described as the new her.

2. **Pick products with more than one use.** This will help you achieve your first goal of limiting exposure while also reducing packaging waste. There are so many uses for individual products. Next time you want to remove your makeup, try some organic olive oil from your cupboard or use your face cream. Shampoo works perfectly as body wash. Some face creams serve as wonderful palette perfecters before applying makeup. *Real* handmade superfatted soap works wonders as a shaving cream. A lot of nighttime eye moisturizers/wrinkle-prevention balms can be used around the lips and cuticles. The list goes on. Try out different applications with the products you are currently using. Be careful to read all the warnings first.

3. **Choose products with a shorter list of ingredients.** More does not necessarily mean better. A lot of what is on a label is either bad for you or is there for show. By choosing products that use fewer ingredients, you will reduce both your exposure to toxins and the damage caused during the manufacture of the product.

4. **Forget about what the label/packaging looks like.** What the bottle says and looks like has nothing to do with performance. Don't let a pretty package sell you; tell yourself the truth. Look for products that use the least amount of packaging possible. Overuse of packaging is a waste of our planet's resources and a strain on our landfills. Also, any company that is willing to forgo the extra sale it will inevitably make with packaging is making a statement and taking active steps to reduce waste.

5. **Don't be sold by name-dropping.** Nostalgia sells products. I often hear, "I use Chanel No. 5, just like my grandmother did," or "I can only use Tide—it reminds me of home." Consumers also relate to major names: "It's Prada face cream, so it has to be

good"; "Johnson & Johnson makes it, so it's safe"; "It cost a hundred dollars for half an ounce, so I know it's good." Let go of any and all preconceived notions and allow yourself to inspect everything and form a nonbiased perspective. You might still wear your grandmother's perfume or buy the hundred-dollar face cream, but first unmask your products and let yourself see the naked truth. This is the only way to really be in charge and make choices based on knowledge rather than nostalgia or marketing.

6. **Make your own criteria for what is acceptable, and stick with them.** One way to do this is to make a list of the top ingredients that you will not put on your skin and find products that do not contain them. Your list could be two or twenty—what counts is that it makes you feel safe and comfortable. Empower yourself and send a message to manufacturers that you purchase products from.

7. **Get intimate with your products.** Look at the products you are using now and read the ingredient lists. Look up any ingredient you do not know and decide whether you want to continue to use it on your body. Take a look beyond what the label says and look inside your products to decide whether they're as beautiful inside as the mask they're hiding behind.

8. **Resist the urge to buy.** Stay away from the beauty aisles. If you have products that you like and that fit your chemical-free criteria, resist the urge to purchase more. When I do my chemical-free makeover, the first thing I notice is just how many products we all have and how many new ones we try. There is always a new exciting miracle cream on the market, but you simply do not need it. Stick with products you know and love and with those whose ingredients you are familiar. Just by curbing your impulse purchases, you will lessen your exposure, save money, and reduce waste.

9. **Switch to mineral makeup.** Even the most harmful mineral makeup has fewer chemicals than most liquid foundations and

pressed powders. There is a large array of mineral makeups on the market, and many are completely chemical-free.

10. **Understand ingredient lists.** Ingredients should be listed in order of most to least. This helps you determine how much of any ingredient is in the product. Many people insist on synthetic fragrances in their products. There are some scents you cannot make naturally. Synthetic fragrance can be blended with essential oils to reduce the amount used. On some labels, fragrance will be listed toward the top, while on others it will be listed closer to the bottom.

Just by following these ten simple rules, you will make a big difference. If you can't make all of these changes, start with one, because even one step makes a difference. Being a label detective is a never-ending project. There is always more we can learn.

Ten Simple Toxic-Exposure Rules to Live By

The following are some quick rules that can help us reduce our exposure to toxins:

1. Use smaller amounts of product.

2. Buy products with understandable ingredient lists.

3. Buy in bulk or with the least amount of packaging.

4. Don't trust the words on the front of the bottle; read the ingredients list.

5. Don't trust the salesperson; get the information yourself.

6. Avoid products about which you are unsure.

7. Call companies and ask questions if you have any concerns about their products; don't be afraid to pester.

8. Babies do not need a cupboard full of products; buy less.

9. Create change by giving clean products as gifts.

10. Make a pocket guide for yourself and carry it with you when shopping.

The Top Ten Products to Avoid, Scrutinize, or Use Less Of

The products on the list are chosen for different reasons. Some are known to be the most toxic, some are problematic due to the extent of exposure, and others have toxic ingredients that do not show up on the labels. There are many products that contain dangerous ingredients that are not required to be listed on the product (see the sidebar for an example). To be safe, the following ten products should be avoided, carefully researched, or used less frequently:

1. powder containing talc

2. nail polish (nearly 70 percent of nail polishes tested contained high levels of a chemical named DBP [dibutyl phthalate])

3. deodorant and antiperspirant

4. baby shampoo

5. bubble bath

6. hair dye

7. petroleum-based products

8. makeup

9. makeup primers made with silicone or other "-cone" products, such as dimethicone or cyclomethicone

10. baby wipes

The contaminant 1,4-dioxane—cited as a probable carcinogen by the U.S. Environmental Protection Agency and an animal carcinogen by the National Toxicology Program—is all-too common in most cosmetics brands. Product tests released by author and researcher David Steinman found 1,4-dioxane in more than twelve best-selling brands of shampoo and bubble bath. It even appears in some organic brands as well. Unfortunately, this is a clear-cut example of what hidden dangers lurk in your products that are not listed on the label. Because 1,4-dioxane is a common contaminant in ingredients used in body care,

(cont'd.)

the FDA does not require that it be listed as an ingredient on product labels.

The Top Ten Ingredients to Avoid

So you don't have to carry a stack of reference books everywhere you go, use this simple list while you're at the store to avoid the top ten worst offenders in bodycare:

1. **parabens** (parabens, used as preservatives, are taking a lot of heat and getting a bad rap for good reasons, but if a product has had parabens removed, make sure that they have not been replaced with an equally bad or worse preservative)

2. **formaldehyde** (The following ingredients contain formaldehyde, may release formaldehyde, or may break down into formaldehyde: 2-bromo-2-nitropropane-1,3-diol, diazolidinyl urea, DMDM hydantoin, imidazolidinyl urea, quaternium-15)

3. **phthalates** (not listed on label, found in fragrance and other ingredients. However, a lot of companies are starting to indicate that their products are "phthalate-free")

4. **diethanolamine (DEA) and triethanolamine (TEA)**

5. **diazolidinyl urea and imidazolidinyl urea**

6. **sodium lauryl/laureth sulfate; ammonium laureth sulphate** (as with parabens, these are getting a lot of heat, while some of their substitutes are equally bad or worse, such as phenoxyethanol, and sodium lauryl sarcosinate)

7. **propylene glycol**

8. **PVP/VA copolymer**

9. **nanoparticles**

10. **synthetic fragrance**

In terms of consumer (that means you) safety, this is possibly the most important list in the book. Make a copy and carry it with you when you go shopping. You can also download this list and all of Appendix C, "Toxic Ingredients List," from www.hunterhouse.com.

Whenever new customers walk into Sumbody, we explain that our products are all natural, and invariably they respond with, "Oh yeah, that's great; I only use all-natural products." Then they tell us about this great product (which we are usually familiar with), and I realize that they mean they use only products that *claim* to be all natural. Unfortunately, this does not mean the product is truly natural. It is a shame that these people are scammed into making bad choices. Consumers have a right to honest, accurate, and freely available information on all the products they are considering.

Chapter 3

Sell You,
Not Tell You

Image is what
the cosmetics industry
sells through its products,
and it's up to the consumer
to believe the claims or not.

— JOHN BAILEY, PHD,
DIRECTOR OF FDA'S OFFICE
OF COSMETICS AND COLORS,
FROM AN ARTICLE IN THE
MAY–JUNE 1998 **FDA CONSUMER**

The following section is an in-depth look at the techniques companies use to both drive sales and make the consumer think something about the product that may not be true.

Driving Sales

Thick, pink plastic spheres of shampoo and tall undulating bottles of face cream with silk-screened figures of women adorn the aisles of stores from CVS to Sephora. A company has about a three-second window to get you to pick a product off a shelf, with another five or so seconds to get you to purchase it. In order to convince you to buy their products, most manufacturers spend more money on creating a "look" and a "hook" for the packaging of a product than they do on the actual ingredients.

But the marketing goes deeper than the label. Companies are trying to hook you with the latest buzz. Consider grapefruit. If grapefruit is in, you'll see articles and huge ads in magazines touting the miracles of grapefruit and building the desire for grapefruit products in the consumer's mind. Companies know this and want to sell their products, so they market products as containing some amount of grapefruit. Unfortunately, the desire to market something as containing some amount of grapefruit does not always lead to a product that contains enough grapefruit to have an effect on the quality of the product. In my business, I have the privilege of being able to talk with many contract manufacturers and chemists. One told me that he was manufacturing and packaging a product for a well-known brand that claimed five active ingredients. Out of the four thousand gallons he manufactured, five grams, about the size of a nickel, of these ingredients were the active ingredients—that comes out to a quantity the size of one nickel in the amount of product it would take to fill about ten average-sized hot tubs.

Unfortunately, this tactic is not unique to this company—most companies do the same thing. Label claims are just that—claims to make a product seem appealing. There is no guideline as to how much of a listed ingredient is actually in the product. Ingredients are required to be listed in order of decreasing volume, but because 75 to 95 percent of most lotions, creams, shampoos, and other personal-care products is water, the first two ingredients can make up virtually the entire product, while the next twenty ingredients are present in miniscule quantities. Consequently, in many cases the minute quantities of these active ingredients have virtually no effect on the product's efficacy. If we compare the results of a grapefruit product to an alfalfa product and to a chocolate product, there will be, at most, a tiny difference, but people will still continue to buy whatever product is being buzzed about at that time. Of course, some companies do use enough of an active ingredient to make a difference, and in this case it matters which active ingredient they're using. However, these companies are not necessarily the ones that are charging upwards of two hundred dollars a bottle. You might think that the more you pay for a product, the better it will be, but price does not generally have anything to do with quality. And for those companies that are not using a noticeable amount of a particular active ingredient, as soon as the buzz about an ingredient dies down, they discontinue that product, wait to hear the new buzz about the next hot product, and then they put that exact body wash back on the shelf, only this time it contains less than a drop of "pomegranate" extract and features a label extolling the miracles of that fruit.

Another common trick used by many manufacturers (both small and large, natural and not) is leaving the extract or active ingredient listed on the label out of the finished product entirely. If they are out of green-tea extract or vitamin C, they do not hold up production, they run the product anyway. There is no agency testing every type of product, and companies are allowed a grace period to change labels, so the ingredients inside the product do not have to match the label. Companies can have an ingredient on the label that is not in the product, they just cannot have anything in the product that is not on the label (for many reasons, one being allergies and other possible reactions).

I know many chemists, manufacturers, and companies who think I am absolutely nutty because I will not run a product unless we have information about absolutely everything in the product. Manufacturers have told me they have, at times, left a certain ingredient out to cut costs, or that customers have requested leaving out some active ingredients for the same reason. This is commonplace.

The old adage "Don't judge a book by its cover" is literal advice in this industry. From the inception of a product to its selling point, given the three-second window companies have to hook you as you walk down the store aisle, money is poured into making the product covers appealing. A chemist who used to work for a major cosmetics company told me he was surprised that there was about a 15:1 ratio between employees in marketing and those in research and development. This means there could be thirty people trying to market a product that only two people have formulated.

To illustrate this point, I pulled out several ads from a national magazine and contrasted their claims with the ingredients in their products. One soap claimed to be 99.72 percent natural. This sounds great—what could be the harm of 0.28 percent? But remember, probably up to 90 percent of this product is water. This leaves 9.72 percent of natural ingredients. Unfortunately, there is no industry regulation for the word *natural*—it is absolutely meaningless. It can mean anything the company wants it to mean.

The next ad I picked was for a major brand that is sold in Wal-Mart, Target, and Safeway, among other outlets. This ad contained a small logo of a panda bear and the words "We are pleased to make an annual donation of at least $100,000 to the World Wildlife Fund." To the average consumer, this is a huge amount of money, and to the World Wildlife Fund it is a considerable donation, but to the company it is a cheap ad. The full-page ad cost the company about $20,000, and it runs one each week. To the company this donation is just another form of marketing. The company makes more money by donating this hundred grand to WWF than it would if it didn't make the donation.

Another ad, this time in the form of a label, featured shampoo in a tube, with the entire tube covered with a picture of luscious red raspberries. The berries look sweet and tantalizing—how could they not be good for your hair? But this is a leap in logic. The company wants you to see something appealing and assume it is good for your hair, yet nowhere on the packaging or in the ad does it tell you anything about how raspberries offer a benefit. It turned out not to matter, because when I looked at the label, raspberries accounted for less than 1 percent of the product's ingredients. At this low concentration, raspberries are not effective in any way.

I chose these three products because each one evokes an emotional response in the consumer's mind. We think, "Oh, it's natural; it must be good for me," or we say to ourselves, "What a great company!" when we see the WWF contribution, or "Oh, raspberries are so tasty, how fresh and luxurious" when we see the pictures of raspberries. This is not a coincidence—these images and claims were chosen to evoke those very responses and to sell you a product that has nothing to do with nature, humanitarianism, or luxury. Labels do not convey the quality or effectiveness of a product.

If They Say It, It Must Be True

A farm that grows food that is certified as organic must undergo a strict process of regulation. Unfortunately, there is no criteria for the beauty industry to adhere to in order to use the term *organic*. In effect, this means that *organic*, just like the word *natural*, can mean whatever a company wants it to mean. Neither of these words have legal definitions in the beauty industry. This is confusing because consumers are inclined to attach the ethos of certified organic food to organic body products. Unfortunately, the Food and Drug Administration (FDA) does not preapprove labels. Its rules only prohibit therapeutic claims on labels of products that do not contain drugs: The agency does not even mention the terms *natural* and *organic*. Therapeutic claims are things like SPF (sun protection factor) or "removes wrinkles." Companies easily skirt this regulation problem by using terms such as "sun cream" and "age-defiant." The result is that the companies trying to sell the products are the ones making the definitions for the words *natural* and *organic*. Even if a company has a working definition for these terms, it may not be in line with your definition. Because there is no standard, there is no way to know which definition a company is using. Some companies may have no definition at all and may simply use these terms as a marketing scheme. However, there are companies that recognize this problem and are working to rectify it. Dr. Bronner has sued ten cosmetics and bath-and-body companies, including Kiss My Face, Avalon Organics, Stella McCartney America, Estée Lauder (which sells Aveda products), Nature's Gate, Ecocert, and Hain Celestial Group (which sells Jasön products), accusing them of using misleading labeling by calling their products organic yet using petroleum-based ingredients. However, there are responsible companies trying to make a difference—they just don't constitute a majority...yet.

Another issue in deciphering a label is that even if you know exactly what ingredients are in a product, you will not know exactly what it is doing to you. I have been at forums where cosmetic chemists engage in heated arguments about those who advocate parabens and those that say they are harmful. There are so many conflicting definitions of what is natural and safe that it seems impossible to reach a consensus. My philosophy is that if it is questionable, do not use it. Parabens have estrogen-like properties, and they have been detected in breast tumors. Though this does not prove a link between parabens and breast cancer, it certainly provides enough evidence to mark them as questionable.

Since 1999 the European Union has prohibited the use of phthalates in children's toys. However, the Cosmetic Ingredient Review (CIR), established in 1976 by the Cosmetic, Toiletry & Fragrance Association (CTFA) with support of the U.S. Food and Drug Administration and the Consumer Federation of America to thoroughly review and assess the safety of ingredients used in cosmetics in an open, unbiased, and expert manner and publish the results in peer-reviewed scientific literature, conducted a study stating phthalates were safe (CFSAN, 2008). Amid the many conflicting studies, the case was closed, and now, six years later, the evidence against phthalates is growing, and the CIR has decided not to reopen the study. In another study, published in 2008 in the journal *Pediatrics*, Dr. Sheela Sathyanarayana, from the University of Washington, Seattle, and colleagues measured the levels of nine different phthalate breakdown products in urine from the diapers of 163 infants aged two to twenty-eight months. All of the urine samples contained at least one phthalate at measurable levels, and 81 percent of the samples had measurable amounts of seven or more phthalates. The presence of these phthalates in the urine is a direct result of the use of creams, lotions, and other baby products that contain phthalates. The supposed watchdog organization of the cosmetic industry is unwilling to further investigate a substance that is questionably harmful and found in babies' urine. "At this time, we do not know what the potential long-term health effects might be, but there is a large body of animal studies to suggest developmental and reproductive toxicity (from phthalates) and a few human studies with changes in health outcomes as well," according to remarks by Dr. Sathyanarayana.

Many chemists will say that there is not enough research supporting claims of a substance's harmful effects. To that I say okay, take it off the market until we have conclusive evidence one way or another, and then bring it back if the substance is found to not be harmful. We lose nothing by taking an ingredient off the market, but we risk everything by continuing to sell it.

Some companies use sneaky tricks to make you assume a product is organic, without making an outright claim that the product is organic. Consider the shampoo company Simply Organic. This is just the company's name—the company does not say that its products are organic. However, most consumers will see a name like that of this company and understandably assume the product is organic—why else would it be named Simply Organic? The tagline reads "with olive leaf extract from the tree of life." This claim sounds amazing—who wouldn't want organic extracts from the tree of life? As I turned the bottle around to read the ingredients list, I noticed that only one of the twenty-one ingredients listed was called organic. Not only are the claims in the company name and in the tagline misleading—remember there is no industry standard for what it means to be organic—but the organic ingredient was honey. I thought that we were at least looking for organic olive leaf extract. Organic honey in a bath product is not the same thing as organic honey from the grocery store.

This seems counterintuitive, especially since honey is a food product; however, because it is not intended for consumption in this case, the FDA standards do not apply. The name of the company is misleading and meaningless because there is no standard for organic body care. In fact, of the first six ingredients, three of them are not only clearly not organic, but they are also at the top of my list of ingredients to avoid (see page 32).

The one exception to the lack of a definition for *organic* is a product that is "certified organic." This is a good sign, but don't stop here. Look for the name of the organization that certified the product and its criteria. Then you will know if your definition fits its definition, and you will know whether you are getting what you expect.

What's on Aisle Seven?

What is really in the bottle of the average personal-care product, and what do we know about its effects?

In my quest to determine just that, I chose to examine products that are, above all, common and readily available, products that can be found in any house.

Sadly, I could have chosen almost any product, since I knew that when you break them down, they are very much the same. On the inside, they all look alike; whether it was a hundred-dollar anti-aging face cream, or a five-dollar drugstore version, the ingredients did not differ that much. This made one thing clear. Since they are all so similar, I should start with products that sell the most and are most accessible regardless of consumers' location or income. So I set off to the store to see where it would lead me.

Walking down the aisle of my local drugstore, I spotted a bottle of Suave body wash. Up front on the label was the confusing, and all-too-common, "natural" claim. The unsubtle picture of a coconut and the claim that the product was filled with its wonderful extract was hardly unique either. What struck me was a little girl with her mother shopping in the same aisle I was inspecting. The girl was drawn to the sexy bottle and alluring picture, while her mother proclaimed its "natural" goodness. This was just the reaction the professionals behind the brand were predicting. On the front panel, used to grab the passersby—the people not married to their favorite brand but who instead hunt the shampoo aisles looking for products that will sweep them away with a promise of true bliss—were some of my of my favorite catchphrases: "pampering body wash" and "tropical coconut." No doubt the young girl had visions of beaches, the sweet smell of coconut, and summertime pleasures; the mother was thinking of health, pampering, relaxation, and being whisked away in her shower. I could understand how they had been misled.

I got to know many people in the personal-care aisle while researching for this book, and their confusion was all the same. Some thought they knew what *natural* was, and others had no idea about it. What they all had in common was an interest in knowing and a desire to make healthier choices.

What really is in this bottle of Suave body wash? There are ingredients that are linked to cancer and complications with reproduction, other harmful toxins, untested chemicals, fragrance, and penetration agents, to name a few.

In reading the label, I cannot understand what is natural here. As far as I can tell, the Suave body wash does not meet any natural standards. It is literally a chemical soup. It contains propylene glycol and tetrasodium EDTA, penetration enhancers that alter the skin structure, allowing other chemicals to penetrate deeper into the skin, increasing the amounts of the other chemicals that reach the bloodstream. As well as being used for everything from creams to cleansers and bubble bath to hair mousse, propylene glycol is also used as a paint solvent, in antifreeze, and as a deicing solution for boats, cars, and aircraft. In January 1991 the American Academy of Dermatologists released a review on propylene glycol, stating that it had been shown to have severe adverse health effects; to cause contact dermatitis, kidney damage, and liver abnormalities; to inhibit skin-cell growth and damage cell membranes; and to cause skin rashes, dry skin, and surface damage.

The entire ingredient list from the back label reads:

◇ water

◇ ammonium lauryl sulfate: The *Journal of the American College of Toxicology* notes that ammonium lauryl sulfate has a "degenerative effect on the cell membranes because of its protein denaturing properties." Additionally, "High levels of skin penetration may occur at even low use concentration." Even the Cosmetic Ingredient Review (CIR) panel, an organization one would think would be vigilant about protecting us from harmful ingredients, states that ammonium lauryl sulfate "appears to be safe in formulations designed for discontinuous, brief use followed by thorough rinsing from the surface of the skin." Most people use soap daily, and the truth is, no one knows what the true effect of long-term exposure to body soap is. I find myself asking why one would want to clean oneself with a product that is safe only when washed off completely and not left on the body for any amount of time. What happens if you take baths or bathe your children with it? You rinse it from your body, but then you soak in it. This situation does not even meet the CIR's generous guidelines. What are our children soaking in? I looked at a bubble bath while I was in the aisle, and it was even worse; it contained ammonium laureth sulfate.

◇ ammonium laureth sulfate: Ammonium laureth sulfate provides a foaming quality that allows for better distribution of the product while washing or while brushing your teeth. When you rinse it off skin, the area will be clean, but it also will have lost moisture from the top layers. In people with any kind of skin disorders—acne, eczema—it will cause an outbreak of that disorder.

Now that the company's product has dried out your skin, it provides a lotion to moisturize your body. Brilliant marketing. The moisturizer is also filled with stuff that dries your skin so you need to apply it more and more frequently. The following list identifies some of these questionable ingredients:

◇ cocamidopropyl betaine (has been indicated as a skin irritant and to cause allergic reactions)

◇ fragrance (has also been indicated as a skin irritant and to cause allergic reactions)

◇ coconut (*Cocos nucifera*) extract (but what is it extracted from?)

◇ cocamide MEA (believed to anesthetize the eyeball, used as a detergent for cleaning cars, trucks, and other vehicles using commercial washing equipment; there are serious contamination concerns)

◇ PEG-5 cocamide (according to the Skin Deep website, this ingredient may be contaminated with impurities linked to cancer and toxicity of one or more biological systems, such as the reproductive and cardiovascular systems)

◇ propylene glycol (see above)

◇ polyquaternium-10 (limited studies and safety information)

◇ glycol stearate (no known hazards)

◇ ammonium chloride (corrodes metal; is linked to cancer, organ system toxicity, and irritation to eyes, skin, respiratory system, and gastrointestinal tracts)

◇ tetrasodium EDTA (nonreproductive-organ toxicity; irritation to skin, eyes, and lungs; enhances skin absorption of other chemicals)

◇ etidronic acid (linked to endocrine disruption, organ system toxicity, and developmental/reproductive toxicity)

◇ methylchloroisothiazolinone (harms the immune system and nonreproductive organ systems)

I'm sure Suave is aware of the growing concerns about the chemicals in cosmetics—its marketing angle tells me so—but it has not yet made the leap to changing what is in the bottle. As studies take place and awareness grows, I hope companies such as this one will make that leap.

The bottle of Suave body wash cost $1.99 for twelve ounces—that is too amazing to be true! At Sumbody, I pay more than that for my bottle, label, raw goods, and filling (i.e., having the bottle filled) of my body wash. The parent company of Suave, Unilever, had fifty billion dollars in sales in 2004. These are sales they do not want to lose, and if these sales figures were affected by consumer preference, the company would change its use of ingredients.

Suave is not alone. These same ingredients live in products sold in better department stores, boutiques, and health-food stores. This commonly used body wash is just one example of what almost every other product looks like. Each has its own story—pampering, rejuvenating, healing, age-defying—and its own cast of characters—tetrasodium EDTA, propylene glycol—but inside, they are all the same stuff.

It is almost too upsetting to think about baby-care products. There is no doubt that babies and children, because their bodies and immune systems are still developing, are much more vulnerable to toxins. Children's skin is thinner and more absorbent than the skin of adults. This means children's skin serves as less of a barrier to toxic chemicals and allows more toxins into their bloodstream. Eczema, allergies, rashes, and skin sensitivities are on the rise, as is early introduction to "baby personal-care products." Clearly, this is a group of products that needs to be scrutinized. I wanted to look at one of the very best-sellers in baby care, so I chose Johnson's Softwash body wash. On the front of the label was the rave, "Best for baby; best for you."

This baby wash is exposing your child to skin and eye irritants such as cocamidopropyl betaine, acrylates/C10-30 alkyl acrylate crosspolymer, PEG-150 distearate, PEG-80 sorbitan laurate, PEG-14M, and sodium laureth sulphate, all of which can be contaminated with the carcinogens dioxane and ethylene oxide, and hormone disrupters such as parabens. There is nothing that moisturizes the skin—only synthetic polymers (plasticlike substances) like polypropylene terephthalate and polyquaternium-7, which coat it, merely giving the impression of smoothness. This also creates a layer of plastic coating in your baby's pores, causing damage and keeping the other chemicals locked in the skin.

With generations of loyal customers, Johnson & Johnson is a company we have come to know, love, and trust. Many parents shampoo their little ones' heads every night with Johnson's shampoo, just as their parents did for them. It is a bond that's hard to break. Johnson & Johnson means baby care.

The Harms of Phthalates

Phthalates are such a health concern that I could write a chapter on them alone. Almost everyone uses them in some form every day, but don't go hunting for them on your labels—you won't find them there. They are hidden in other ingredients, such as fragrance. They are regulated as toxic pollutants, but it is legal to use them in consumer products. The chemical industry and the federal government have an interesting relationship with phthalates. Phthalates are recognized as toxic substances by the Occupational Safety and Health Administration (OSHA), but companies are free to use unlimited amounts in cosmetics. They are considered hazardous waste and regulated as pollutants in both air and water, yet they go completely unregulated in personal-care products. Under various environmental laws, companies are limited as to how much they can release into the environment each year. Do they record the "spillage" into our personal-care products, or the "transportation" into our bodies? And why does the FDA not require cosmetic manufacturers to test their products for safety or limit the amount of these harmful ingredients, which it monitors in other industries, that are used in personal-care products?

A partial list of the adverse effects connected with phthalates includes liver damage; reproductive effects such as low birthweight, decreased pregnancies, decreased sperm count; birth defects; and endocrine disruption, which can lead to cancer, birth defects, immune-system depression, and developmental problems in children.

Hunting for Chemicals

Even more interesting to me was trying to find information about these products from chemical suppliers or to obtain samples of the ingredients themselves. We don't use these chemicals at Sumbody, but I wanted the Material Safety Data Sheets (MSDSs) on ingredients I list as harmful in the book, and being in the industry, I have access to chemical manufacturers. My purchasing agent could not believe how difficult it was trying to obtain these raw ingredients, even to have samples and MSDSs sent. Some companies have them but will not sell them individually, only in a blend. These companies did not want to answer her questions and were wary about selling their ingredients to a company that didn't already use them—it was so different from ordering shea butter or cocoa butter. Yet anyone can go to the grocery store and buy hundreds of products filled with these ingredients! At first I thought it was because we are a small company that we had such a difficult time getting assistance, but then I realized many small companies' products contain chemicals. Yet most of these companies are not making their own products, no matter what they say—they're made in large labs with access to these chemicals. This experience only affirmed my belief that these chemicals are not meant for our skin.

Upon returning home from my shopping trip, I was holding my body wash and baby wash, wondering what to do with them. I thought of the hazardous-waste disposal days we have in our town. These are the designated times when we can bring our toxic household substances—paint, paint solvents, oven cleaners, and used motor oil (stuff we know to be harmful to the environment if it pollutes groundwater and/or the atmosphere)—to the dump for safe disposal. Some of the very same ingredients that are in these household products are in your personal-care products. Cresol, formaldehyde, sodium lauryl sulfate, glycols, nitrates/nitrosamines, and sulfur are found in many shampoos. Butane propellants are in hair sprays. Aerosol propellants, ammonia, triclosan, and aluminum chlorohydrate are in deodorants. Phenol, fragrance, and artificial coloring make it into just about everything, as do petroleum products, propylene glycol, and numerous other toxins listed in the household hazardous waste disposal list.

Should I save my unused bottle of shampoo and body wash for hazardous-waste disposal day, and dispose of them under the observation of all my curious neighbors and friends? After all I knew now, knowledge that allows me to make choices about my own life, I felt so powerful. I realize that making small changes is all that is needed to make a difference. Significant change can start with this small bottle when it is multiplied by all of us who are tired of being "cleaned" with toxins. We can cease purchasing products that are destructive to ourselves, our children, and our environment and say yes to using our dollars to make a difference.

Chapter 4

The Conventional Product

The Process

This chapter explains the cycle a typical, conventional product follows from concept to shelf.

Concept to Shower

A crazy scientist, a lab coat, the search to create the perfect lotion.... Unfortunately, this is not the scenario that actually takes place when a new product is created. Marketers, not chemists, formulate products. Products are formulated in order to be sold, not to solve problems. Marketers create the concept of a product, including the newest buzz-worthy ingredient, march it down to the chemist's office, and ask what it will take to get a product that fits their specs. Then the chemist gets to tangle with the specifics of how to create this product. Raw-ingredient manufacturing companies promote their newest ingredients, and the chemist might add a new concept, but ultimately the decision resides with the marketers and whether or not an idea will sell. Marketers are constantly watching for the next market trend. This means looking at the population and analyzing data to decide whether to create baby products or antiwrinkle creams. Marketers predict everything from the soon-to-be-hottest scent to the tagline (e.g., "natural"), packaging, and consistency, and they make sure their new line fits with their prediction regarding the next trend. It is about moving units. Moving units is the most important aspect of marketing. More important than the formula or the quality of a product is the packaging, look, and tagline that sell it.

Generally, the manufacture of the actual product is the last step in the process of its creation. First the marketers go to the art department and plan the packaging. They go to the copy department and get the text for the label. (You might think that the copywriter would want to feel a product and know exactly what it is before writing selling points and hook lines, but this step often takes place before a product exists. It is kind of like an expectant mother. She has diapers, the nursery, the crib, the clothing, and the name—everything but the baby.) Finally, the marketers have to come up with the price for their product. Some products cost twenty-five cents to produce and are sold for twenty-five dollars. There is no standard markup ratio—it is all about what the market will bear. A company will charge as much as the consumer will pay and on a scale that fits in with their brand image. This means that a brand targeting middle-class women may cost the same to manufacture as a brand targeting older, wealthier women, but the latter product will cost ten times more.

The money being poured into the marketing of products cripples small businesses. They cannot order in increments as large as the huge corporations, so their supplies and packaging will be more expensive. Often smaller companies cannot afford to employ a professional text editor or artist, so they don't have the same edge of being able to grab a consumer's eye on the shelf. They are also working under a smaller profit margin because their materials cost more and their products are sold for less, comparatively speaking. In terms of pricing, most small companies are about mid-range—neither extremely cheap nor outrageously expensive. This means they have less capital, and it is more difficult for them to grow in order to be able to compete with the larger companies.

Sourcing: Raw Ingredients

It is extremely important to know where raw ingredients come from. This means both geographically and in what conditions. Purchasing ingredients from a local business has a much lower environmental impact than purchasing the same ingredients from another continent. Furthermore, you have to consider the conditions under which the product is manufactured. Some companies are more environmentally conscious than others, creating less air and water pollution. Typically, the companies that produce the greatest amount of pollution are the ones that manufacture chemicals. As you've learned by now, many of the same chemicals used in cosmetics are used in motor oil, paint thinners, and a plethora of other products. These are the most dangerous plants where one might work.

This is a part of the decision about where a company decides to purchase its raw ingredients. Companies can choose to support large, polluting companies with poor worker-health standards half a world away or they can choose to be more environmentally responsible by purchasing ingredients from companies with good employee protections. Of course, you can't always get all good or all bad—companies have to balance their priorities.

To give you an idea of the process of creating, processing, and shipping synthetic ingredients, I will use methylparaben as an example. While parabens can be derived from many substances, the cheapest and most widely used is petroleum. Petroleum must be drilled, extracted, refined, turned into mineral oil, and then sent to the manufacturing company to go through a whole set of changes to make it into methylparaben. Not only is this not a sustainable product, it also causes immense strain on the environment. Apart from the known environmental hazards of drilling for oil, the process of turning mineral oil into parabens alone requires numerous chemicals that pose a harm to the workers, releases air pollution, pollutes the surrounding ground and water environment, and creates toxic waste, which even when handled and disposed of properly (which isn't always the case) poses a threat to our health and environment.

Sourcing: Packaging

There are many types of packaging. Cosmetic companies usually spend more money on packaging than they do on what is inside the bottle. And according to Rose Marie Williams, they spend more on television ad space than any other industry (*Townsend Letter*, 2004). Consumers love packaging; it can be cute, spunky, and fun, or it can be elegant and classy; it makes us feel like we're unwrapping a present. The only problem is, the more packaging, the more waste. It leads to overfilled landfills, toxic incinerators, and deforestations. It also has dire consequences stemming from the fact that some paper products leach bleach and some plastic packaging involves petroleum and is nonbiodegradable. Are there any postconsumer products in the packaging? Where was it manufactured? What is it made of? These are only a few of many important considerations for both companies and consumers. As with raw ingredients, it puts more strain on the environment to ship large containers of packaging across a continent than to purchase it nearby. There have been many studies that point out the harmful effects of plastic water bottles leaching chemicals into the water supply. Because many types of beauty packaging are made from the very same plastic as water bottles, those chemicals are leaching into the beauty products as well—and then into the water. Softer plastics tend to leach more toxins than harder plastics. As disgusting as it is to be drinking toxins, it is equally or more disgusting to be slathering them all over our bodies.

The environmental aspect of packaging also makes it more difficult for smaller companies to compete. A representative from a large hotel recently approached me and asked to purchase my company's products for its amenities. At first I thought, "No way," because I did not want to be a part of the thousands of one-ounce bottles that would have to be produced and thrown away. I reconsidered because I realized that at least my products would involve no chemicals, and that would drastically reduce the impact on the environment and personal health. When I looked into buying the bottles, I found that in order to compete, I would have to buy hundreds of thousands at a time. Because the hotel would not come close to consuming all of these, they would have to sit on my shelf until I could sell them to other accounts. This means they would have to be preserved using various synthetic preservatives. I was unwilling to do this. At this point it was clear I couldn't compete. Buying the right number of bottles for what this hotel could use in the course of a year had me paying about nine cents each, without a label or a product. The other companies were selling their finished product for five to twenty-five cents! These weren't only off-brand companies either—some were well-known, well-respected companies. Some of these companies were even having their products mass-produced overseas in an effort to cut costs.

Who Will Sell, Who Will Buy?

Many consumers are willing to believe that enormous companies are harmful and small producers are safe and healthful. Unfortunately, this is not always the case. While I don't know of many truly responsible large companies, I do know that many small companies use harmful toxic synthetic ingredients. However, it is true that larger companies produce more pollution and waste simply because they produce in such high volume. These are the products that are sold at CVS, Safeway, Rite-Aid, Wal-Mart, and other multibillion-dollar chains. Consumers walk by these stores almost every day and shop in them because they are conveniently located and ingrained in our minds. The companies that create products grow fatter, and it becomes increasingly difficult for a small business to compete. So even if a small company is environmentally responsible, its products have a slim-to-zero chance of becoming widely carried and held. Getting into Harvard is nothing in comparison to getting a new brand on the shelf of one of these major stores. And the lucky few companies that are awarded shelf space are often so much more expensive that people will not purchase their products, which then limits the amount of capital these companies have access to, which in turn limits their ability to create more affordable products.

The small companies that survive are quickly slurped up by the large companies. For instance, Stila Cosmetics was bought out by Estée Lauder and then sold to Sun Capital Partners, while Burt's Bees was snapped up by Clorox. The latter is especially interesting. Traditionally, the largest players in the cosmetic industry are the ones buying out the smaller companies. Since cosmetics have become so hot, companies outside of the industry, like Clorox, have started buying them as a profitable investment. When a company is purchased by another company, it does not necessarily have to decrease in integrity or quality, but there are a few key reasons why it usually does. First, with products being sold on a larger scale, these companies turn to mass production and can stock a product for up to three years before it even ships to a retail outlet. With products sitting around for so long, these large corporations can't risk a consumer getting rancid goods, so they start using stronger and larger quantities of chemical preservatives. Some of these chemicals are harmful. These companies know that at the very least, they can't risk the consumer getting bad goods and knowing for certain it was the fault of the company—

chemical exposure, hazards, and health issues are an entirely different story. Synthetic alternatives are also more widely available and affordable than natural ingredients, allowing companies to produce cheap products on a large scale. A company using orange essential oil cannot afford to have the price triple if orange growers have a bad crop. Because chemicals are not a commodity, if a company uses a lab-produced fragrance, it does not take this type of risk. Essentially, it all comes down to price.

How Far-Reaching Is the Exposure?

Chemical pollution begins with the production of raw ingredients. Energy is employed in vast amounts; air, rivers, lakes, and soil are polluted; and crops are harvested without proper consideration of biodiversity or sustainability. Many companies use petrochemicals such as petroleum jelly and mineral oil, which deplete natural resources. Compared with agricultural crops such as apricots, pistachios, and olives, which can be grown in a sustainable fashion, petrochemicals are not renewable. Shipping to a manufacturing plant adds more pollution to the tab. Manufacturers use even more electricity and produce similar waste and pollution. Often ingredients are subjected to animal testing, which means that animals are raised, housed, and fed for the sole purpose of being forced to consume potentially harmful chemicals, which often results in cancer, decreased sperm count, loss of basic survival skills, and death. And so many ingredients have been shown to cause these effects in animals before being released on the market that we have to wonder what exactly is the purpose of this testing. At what point is a product deemed unmarketable? Does it have to cause immediate death? It appears so.

After testing, the product is shipped again before it sits on the shelf of a store in your neighborhood, where you purchase it and bring it home. As you shower, your body absorbs the chemicals, and excess chemicals are washed down the drain and released into our waterways. You throw the bottle away, and it ends up in a landfill somewhere as a testament to our gluttony. The tab keeps on growing, and so far, no one is volunteering to pay it.

≳ **Things to Keep in Mind When Choosing to Change Your Beauty Habits**

1. Chemicals in products can adversely affect our health.

2. Chemicals from products pollute our environment.

3. Excess packaging creates waste.

4. Petroleum-based products use up nonrenewable resources.

5. Advertising creates false images of how we should look, adversely affecting self-esteem.

6. Our desire to look beautiful creates a "need" for products beyond reality. Do you really need five face creams?

7. Animal testing is frequently conducted to ensure the safety of these toxic chemicals.

8. Humans are exposed to harmful chemicals during the manufacturing of products.

9. Our landfills and waterways are contaminated with residue from cosmetic chemicals.

10. Our unborn babies receive cosmetic chemicals transmitted through their umbilical cords.

Chapter 5

The Natural Product

The Process

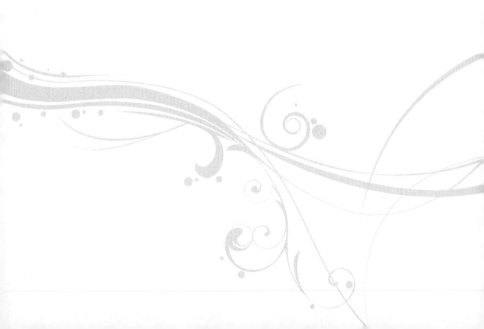

This chapter explains the cycle a natural product follows from concept to shelf.

Concept to Shower

If the producer of a natural body-care product is a large company with large-company resources, it will use the same advantages the large chemical companies have. This means marketing, searching for the "buzz" ingredient, packaging, and everything else that goes into the process of selling a brand. However, none of the companies I have seen that produce truly "natural" products have this kind of financial capability. As a small manufacturer myself, I would benefit from those resources, which would enable me to create a healthful alternative that could compete with the status quo. Natural companies search for the most stylish packaging they can afford. There are two types of packaging—stock packaging and custom packaging. Stock packaging is available to anyone, and often you see many of the same types of containers on the market. You can dress stock packaging up by using silk-screening, labels, and other creative touches, but it can only become so cute. Custom packaging can involve any shape, size, color, or material, and I have seen some fabulous examples. Of course, custom packaging is more expensive, with higher minimums. Large companies—natural or not—can afford to create custom packaging, while smaller companies rely on creativity to dress up the stock packaging that is readily available without minimums. I often wish I could have a different-colored lid or differently shaped bottle.

Another main difference between the conventional and natural processes is that the natural companies do not have the resources or clout to create a theme and a buzz. They try to use buzz ingredients and hop on the trends, but most importantly, a small natural company's theme stays true to its concept. For example, a company might be paraben-free or use honey or bee products, and will be best off sticking to its own concept rather than trying to latch on to an industry theme.

The natural companies strive to target the same consumer base as the chemical companies, but they do not have the same capability. They don't have the resources to create snazzy packaging that will attract a teen's attention or the money to hire market analysts. In order to woo a teen, for example, a small company will try to convince her that it is more effective and sustainable to use natural products and will try to gain customers through the company ethos and brand concept rather than through outrageous packaging in the shape of a multifaceted gem. In addition, many smaller companies don't have the resources to target all strata of society. This means they might only have a line of products for women, or they might only target adults.

Just like chemical companies, natural companies set the prices for their products according to what the market will bear. Unfortunately, it costs a company an obscene amount more to produce a product naturally than synthetically. Right off the bat, a small company will have to pay more for its raw ingredients because it will not be able to afford to purchase a large-enough quantity to receive the bulk discount or economy-scale pricing. It will have to pay more for packaging, labeling, and production, too. In many cases, stock packaging for a small company will cost more than custom packaging for a large company. But this company cannot afford custom packaging minimums. Labels present the same problem—not only is there a large start-up fee, but smaller companies don't order in large-enough quantities to receive economy-of-scale prices. It costs more for a small company to manufacture a product because in most cases it cannot afford an in-house chemist. This means all the formulating has to be farmed out to auxiliary companies, which charge more for the same work than it would cost to do the work in-house. Often the formulas do not even belong to the company because the co-packers (companies that package products for a number of different smaller companies that cannot afford their own packaging equipment) make money by owning the formula. A formula can cost anywhere between five and fifty thousand dollars, and most companies don't have the money to buy the formulas they use. It is also more advantageous for a co-packer to own all of the formulas and use a similar formula for many companies in order to reach its own minimums for economy of scale. Beauty companies far outnumber co-packers, which means that one co-packer often sells nearly the same product to hundreds of companies in order to reduce costs and maximize profits.

A product might cost five cents to produce and sell for fifteen dollars. This price has nothing to do with the quality of the product and more to do with how much a consumer within the company's targeted consumer base will be willing to pay for that product. A consumer walking down the aisle at CVS will not be willing to shell out sixty bucks for a face cream, so the companies whose products are sitting on the shelf in CVS will have to price their products accordingly. On the other hand, a consumer strolling through Saks Fifth Avenue in New York probably will not purchase a face cream for less than sixty dollars for fear of the product being inferior.

A while ago, a woman came into my store to inquire about our face oil. It is an exquisite product containing oils from around the world, infused together in a bottle to perfectly complement one's body's natural oils; it moisturizes the skin and maintains natural health through the use of ingredients from antioxidants to vitamin A. The woman was excited about the product and asked for the price. I told her, a one-ounce bottle costs about thirty dollars. Hesitation flitted across her face, and she replaced the bottle onto the shelf. No matter what I said at first, she was convinced it could not be as good as it sounded because it didn't cost at least ninety dollars. I told her about how all the products are priced according to what the market will bear, and that the price doesn't mean the product is "cheap" and ineffective. Eventually she was convinced, purchased the face oil, and returned several weeks later to buy five more bottles for her girlfriends. Just as "cheap" products can be amazingly effective, many expensive products are virtually worthless. In a Saks Fifth Avenue store, I saw a daily moisturizing kit that featured a dab of cream, which you push out of a foil container, for use each day; it retailed for almost two hundred dollars a month. I itched to know what was inside of it. With the help of a chemist, I dissected the cream and came up with an estimate for what it would have cost the manufacturer. Each day's worth of cream cost less than one penny! But if the product sold for a dollar, everyone would assume it was worthless. The power of perception in relationship to price is overwhelming and is in many ways priceless.

Sourcing: Ingredients

Sourcing truly natural ingredients is a vastly different process from sourcing synthetic ingredients because everything comes directly from the earth. This means a company has much less to worry about in terms of environmental and health hazards in the production of raw ingredients. It does not mean that the production of these ingredients has no negative impact. Some companies employ sustainable, renewable agricultural practices, while others do not. Some companies are greener in terms of packaging and shipping practices, and some grow higher-quality ingredients than others. Additionally, some products are grown organically, and some are grown using pesticides, which can contain petrochemicals and a slew of other harmful chemicals. But overall, purchasing natural ingredients is much less detrimental to the environment and human health than purchasing chemicals.

To give you an idea of the process for growing, harvesting, processing, and shipping natural ingredients, let's look at jojoba. While it is usually called jojoba oil, the term "oil" is a misnomer because it is much more similar to a liquid wax or a liquid ester than to an oil. It is produced mechanically by pressing jojoba seeds to extract the oil. It is one of the few oils that mimic the exact breakdown of our skin secretions, which makes it ideal for protecting and replenishing skin's moisture. Unlike most synthetic ingredients, jojoba is a sustainable, low-impact crop. It grows wild in Tucson, Arizona, and is easily farmed in California, Argentina, Peru, and Chile. Native to the Sonoran Desert in North America, jojoba is easily grown organically, and even when it is grown conventionally it requires few chemical pesticides. Curious about this property, I called my distributor in Arizona, who told me that not only could she not think of anything that preys on jojoba but also that the seeds contain a natural appetite suppressant to ward off bugs and animals that might otherwise attempt to feast on it. Jojoba requires little to no irrigation, no synthetic processing, and is farmed relatively near my company. This means it causes minimal environmental strain and pollution because the factory does not employ solvents or excess chemicals. The environmental impact would be greater for companies manufacturing products in China or Europe, but jojoba is still one of the best raw ingredients available in terms of environmental impact and benefit to the consumer.

Sourcing: Packaging

When it comes to sourcing packaging for natural products, companies face the same slew of concerns faced by chemical producers. Companies seeking the lowest impact on the environment will choose packaging made from partially postconsumer materials that is produced relatively locally and has environmentally friendly waste, pollution, and energy standards. In addition, they will avoid unnecessary amounts of packaging.

Who Will Sell, Who Will Buy?

A company with stock packaging and ten employees cannot afford a commercial on prime time. Glossy two-page spreads in *Lucky* magazine are a distant fantasy, and billboards in downtown San Francisco belong to a separate world. Distributors and large retail chains know this, and most are unwilling to carry these relatively low-end products. Consumers buy based on comfort. This means the more a consumer is exposed to a brand or idea, the more likely she will purchase those products. It isn't profitable for a store like CVS or Sephora, which carries a variety of beauty-care products from across the price spectrum, to carry a product that does not have the resources to market itself on a large scale. These stores want popular brands that consumers know and are willing to purchase. This leaves the smaller companies in the dust, scrambling for viable alternative marketing schemes. This is where webpages, small stores, and spas come into play. Most of their sales are conducted on a small scale. Small retail stores that carry a variety of products often sell these smaller companies' wares for two reasons. Many larger companies are unwilling to sell to these outlets because they don't have the capacity to move as many units as a CVS or Sephora. These small retailers often have a trained and personalized staff, and they depend on intimacy in customer relations. Consumers can obtain unlimited personal attention and problem solving. This knowledge and attention helps make up for a brand's lack of national clout. But don't discount their potency just because they don't seem to be as well known as the leading brands. Here, hidden in the vastness of product globalization, you'll find some of the most effective and truly natural products on the market.

How Far-Reaching Is the Exposure?

Although manufacturing natural raw ingredients consumes energy, the pollution created is drastically less than that created in the manufacture of synthetic ingredients. In terms of packaging and shipping costs, the environmental impacts are the same, unless a company has sought out environmentally friendly alternatives. The most significant aspect of using a natural product is the decrease in personal and environmental exposure to toxic chemicals. Your skin, hair, and face will look and feel healthier and more vibrant, and the earth will have one less caustic chemical oozing into it.

PART II

Let's Go Comparison Shopping

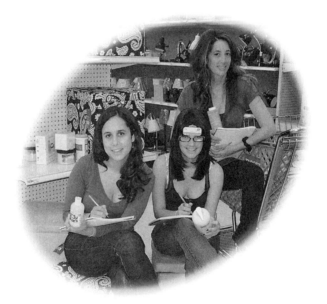

Autumn and Mica help out with market research at Target (equipped with borrowed reading glasses and desks!)

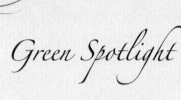

Green Spotlight

Marcia Gay Harden,
Oscar-Winning Actress and Activist

"As an actress, I've had the opportunity to portray many types of people, each one different and each one challenging. When people stop me on the street or in airports, what makes me most proud is when they comment on identifying with a particular character, sharing how it has illuminated something about life for them—a struggle or perhaps a joy.

"In real life, too, we all wear so many different hats. Each challenging. Each amazing. The one that's truly inspiring to me is my role as a mother. Being a mom has informed every choice I make. It makes me want to be wiser, be better, be more informed…not just for my children, but for all children—we are all so connected. I'm trying to guide these little personalities and allow them to be the best possible version of themselves. Really, that's what every parent is trying to do. So I'm educating them. Teaching them about how to live a life that is pure and true and inspiring.

"To live a life that fits those three criteria, I think we have to look at all of our choices and make certain they're ones of integrity and care. So we turn off the lights when we leave a room. We don't leave the water running when we brush our teeth. We drive less. We carpool more. We buy organic everything whenever possible…food, clothes, bedding, even beauty products, like Sumbody's line. Our family is vegetarian (read **Slaughterhouse** by Gail A. Eisnitz), and my ten-year-old daughter is an avid animal-rights activist, so using beauty products that don't test on animals is of paramount importance to us.

"As a family, we do what we can to limit our exposure to potentially harmful chemicals and practices. We do what we can to make sure that our individual choices are in support of the greater good for one another and for our planet. My role as a mother has made me a mediator (breaking up that sibling squabble); a housekeeper (yes, I do shout to pick up those clothes); a caregiver (providing for their futures); and so much more. As we hear on the news about our planet struggling, that we are being exposed to more toxins, and that childhood diseases are on the rise, I've added advocate to my list of roles! It's one I relish and one I know I'll always play…for me, for my family, and for everyone who cares to keep our earth green and our bodies healthy. I find new awareness, change, and hope all around, and I know that with companies like Sumbody, we are on our way to a green century!"

Chapter 6

Dare to Go Bare

Beauty rests on necessities.

— RALPH WALDO EMERSON

Just say yes.

One of our own at Sumbody, who has been with the company for seven years, had no knowledge about the distinctions between or potential effects of chemical and natural products before working for us. In fact, when she saw the body oil I used as the chemical example in this book, she said, "That's what I used when I was growing up." She'd used an array of chemical cocktails and was "happy" with her beauty regimen. Time changes everything. Since working for Sumbody, she has switched to using only our products and has not touched synthetic-based products for quite some time. So I was amazed by her reaction when a spa sent us some samples of a chemical-laden lotion and asked us to come up with a natural alternative.

I made a natural lotion to send to the spa, and before I could label which was the one I had formulated and which was the original lotion sample sent to me, my employee sent one off to the spa. At first I was upset, and I said, "How could you send the lotion without me confirming you were sending our natural version?" Insulted, she exclaimed, "How could I not know?" After years away from chemicals, her skin could tell which one was natural. She said the other felt so bad she could smell the plastic chemicals and had to wash them off immediately. I checked which sample she had sent, and she was right.

When you have only experienced chemical cosmetics, your skin might not know the difference. They may feel wonderful. But once you make the change you can never go back. Your skin will not let you. It is kind of like loving coffee. If each morning you trudge down to the neighborhood 7-Eleven to get your fix, you'll be completely satisfied. But the first time someone hands you an aromatic cup of fresh French-press organic brew, you'll never look at your old coffee the same way.

Natural Results

Raising two daughters in a chemical-dependent, beauty-driven culture can be challenging at best. The media sells them an image they want to achieve, and the cosmetic aisles are filled with products that promise to make their dreams come true.

While I listened to other parents fret over the potential struggles their children might encounter, such as drugs and sex, I had my own list of issues. In my house the drugs we fought over were the ones used in deodorant, nail polish, shampoo, and other personal-care items. My children were raised using alternative products, but when puberty hit they ran to the deodorant aisle at full speed. I lectured and demanded, and we fought over a two-ounce bottle. I realized what they were going through and had complete sympathy; I knew if they felt "protected" from odor and embarrassment, a natural product would be fine with them. Even with their background, they were reluctant to believe that a natural deodorant could work. After several attempts I made them one they liked, and after using it for a period and seeing that it worked, they happily switched.

It is hard for most people to step outside their comfort zone and try something new, especially when it comes to an aspect as fundamental as smelling nice. Truth be told, if you have used a chemical-based antiperspirant or deodorant for years, it takes time for your body to adjust. They clog your pores and set off a signal for your body to produce more sweat. The longer you have used it, the stronger your odor becomes and the more you tend to need it. This is true for a lot of chemical-based products.

The results produced by natural products can be far better than what their chemical rivals offer, but it can take time. It takes time to undo the chemical conflict that your current products have created, to feed and restore your skin, and to show results. You are not eradicating or annihilating acne overnight, you are reducing redness and inflammation, killing the bacteria that causes it, and reducing scarring—things that take time but make a long-term difference. Anyone who has sprained an ankle or had an infection knows it takes time to reduce the swelling or for the infection to heal. We want immediate results, we want to believe we can look ten years younger overnight or wake up acne-free, but results like that are not realistic. In addition, unnaturally speeding up skin repair leads to long-term skin disasters such as redness, pimples, rashes, and accelerated aging.

For those who think natural ingredients cannot be as active, productive, or strong as synthetics, think about what nature has provided. Nature has proven its ability to change and alter everything from our minds, via drugs such as marijuana, tobacco, and peyote, to our health, via products such as antibiotics derived from mold. Nature has proven so powerful that we have outlawed the use of certain plants and herbs because of their effects.

Natural products work by solving the root of problems, whereas chemical products are focused on attacking symptoms. Picture a tree with an infected limb. Conventional and synthetic companies would treat the limb with medicine, wrap it up, and check the progress of its healing. Natural products would focus on the root system of the tree, feeding it and nurturing it so the entire tree will be healthier, allowing the limb to grow stronger and have the capacity to heal itself. Natural products target the underlying issues that cause skin problems, rather than covering up the issues with concealers or killing off the skin with a chemical peel.

Nature Knows Best

In an effort to be healthy we try to eat the best foods we can. Most people would agree that fresh, simple, and unprocessed foods are the most nutritious and the least harmful for us. Some of the same foods that form a healthful diet are vital to healthy skin. Your skin cells function very much like the cells in the rest of your body.

Imagine eating a diet full of synthetic foods. Plastic cereal for breakfast, a sandwich of polymers and fragrance, a chemical soufflé for dinner. Most of us would politely decline. We are told to stay away from foods filled with artificial colors and flavors. In the movie *Super Size Me* we watched a healthy thirty-two-year-old male go from 185 pounds to 210 pounds in one month by eating large amounts of over-processed, synthetic fast foods. In the same way, when we feed our skin junk, it suffers, becoming dry, red, and wrinkled. It takes time for these adverse effects to show up, but when they do, the damage has been done. Naturally, we have all the elements skin needs. Nature provides vitamin C in rose-hip oil, vitamins A and D in carrot oil, and antioxidants in green-tea extracts. Why do we need synthetic alternatives?

I am constantly having to interact with manufacturers' sales reps who are trying to sell me some new chemical miracle ingredient. They tell me that it contains vitamin C in a higher concentration, works for twenty-four hours, or has some other virtue. First, do we really need it to be better? If we get enough vitamin C from rose-hip oil, is it better to have more? Just because something is good for us does not necessarily mean more is better. Take water, for example. Consuming it is vital for our existence, yet consuming too much can kill us. Second, not all vitamin C is created equal. Some is not stable and cannot stay active in lotion, and some is not in a form your skin can easily metabolize.

Without even entering the debate over whether chemical personal-care products are harmful to your health or the environment, you can be sure they are not good for your skin. The $150 super-duper face cream you are buying to reduce wrinkles and keep your skin moist is, unfortunately, only drying it out.

Fear of Commitment

When you are ready to go natural, you can make changes slowly, switching one product at a time, or do it all at once; either way, you have to be committed. It takes time to see the full results, so don't get discouraged. Your skin might go through an adjustment period during which it seems worse. As it starts to detoxify and purge the chemicals from its pores, it might break out, feel dry, or suffer other mild symptoms. Do not get a facial unless you read the labels yourself and know what products are being used. If the products contain chemicals, using them at this point will reverse the progress you're making.

Fear of Change

It might take a few tries to find a brand or product that works for you. Every company should have testers in a store or offer samples. When you switch products it can take a while to get used to the new feel and scent. We can be such creatures of habit that change, even for the best, is hard. Lotions with real oils will feel different at first, perhaps heavier or not so smooth. Some natural brands may use alcohol as their preservative, which can be drying for many types of skin. As with so much in life, it may take time to find what you need, but don't fear it—dive in head first.

Breaking Free of Chemical Dependency

Mineral oils, the most common emollients used in synthetic products, can dry out the under layer of the skin so it loses its ability to moisturize itself and becomes dependent on moisture being constantly replaced from an external source. Mineral oils and their derivatives are occlusive, clogging pores and making it difficult for your skin to breathe. Over time, the oils turn rancid and start forming free radicals, whose effects on the skin are very harmful. Most commercial skin-care products contain silicones, plasticlike substances responsible for the smooth, rich texture you can find in high-end moisturizers. Like mineral oils, silicones and other plasticizers form a layer like a coat of plastic on your skin, preventing it from taking in oxygen and interfering with its ability to expel toxins and absorb nutrients.

Those are some of the adverse effects chemicals have on our skin that we can feel and see, but there are more subtle effects as well. Most bar soaps are detergents that dry out your skin. The dryness makes you want to use lotion. Most lotions contain either alcohol or petroleum-based ingredients, which further dry your skin, causing you to use more of the lotion, which in turn causes even more dryness. Your skin becomes dependent on the very product that is causing the problem you are trying to combat. When you break the dependency there will be a period of adjustment. It will take some time for your body and the new chemical-free products you are using to restore (in this example) moisture levels, allow your body's own moisture to be replenished, and heal your skin. After two to four weeks your skin will no longer be as parched, and you can then use less product to keep it hydrated.

My Findings

In an effort to make truly natural products as accessible as possible, I set out with the goal of finding chains, websites, and widely known brands that fit my criteria for providing a healthful product. I broke these down into three categories: "Good," "Better," and "Best." "Good" is just that, a good alternative, while "Best" contains the least amount of chemicals and synthetics I could find in a product. I was surprised to find that the information I needed to categorize a product as "Good," "Better," or "Best" was not easy to come by. I thought it would be a project that would take four days at most; I would call up a bunch of companies, get a list of the ingredients they use, sort out the information, and create my three lists. When I began calling companies, I found them reluctant to reveal their ingredients. I even asked, "If you are really all natural, why can't I get a copy of your ingredients lists?" I ended up having to literally go to large stores and set up shop with pens, paper, my daughters, and a cart full of beauty products. I invested hundreds of hours in copying labels and researching ingredients. I did the work so you don't have to.

At Sumbody, in order to avoid copycats, I have never posted our ingredient lists online, but anyone can call our store and be told the ingredients in a product. We literally have people walk into our store and say, "I love you guys, I'm gonna knock you off," in just about those words. One day, the manager of a well-known celebrity phoned our office and requested more than two thousand dollars' worth of free product. I explained that we were a small company and could not afford to give away that much product to a single person, to which she replied indignantly, "Do you know who you're speaking with?" I did, but it still was not a wise financial decision to give away all that product. Shortly thereafter, the celebrity himself ordered more than two thousand dollars' worth of product from our website, and months later his wife launched her own line of products. Some of hers were exact replicas of ours, so it was clear to me he'd been ordering the products for market research. I always figured, if they're going to knock me off or use our products for market research, they should at least have to purchase the product.

But as I researched other products, my opinion changed. There is something wrong with a company that touts its all-natural organic product while simultaneously refusing to post ingredients. If a product is that fantastic, its ingredients should be an advertising boost. I decided that I would not compromise the integrity of my brand by hiding my ingredients, so I've decided they're going on the Web—even if it gives copycats a field day. Some companies go so far as to package their products with peel-off tabs that list the ingredients underneath. Many are sealed, so you are really not supposed to tamper with them in the store, but how can you be expected to purchase a product without looking at the ingredients list? I understand there are space issues, especially when working with small products and when having to include lengthy Latin terms on the labels, but companies have to find a way to accommodate visible ingredient lists.

I learned a lot from researching. I have every product I could possibly want in a truly natural form, so it has been a long time since I went out and shopped for other products. This research opened my eyes to the extent companies will go to in order to hide their ingredients. I had to restrain myself from adding "Worst Offender" to my "Good," "Better," "Best" lists because I got so angry about meaningless claims. I don't have an issue with there being chemical products on the shelf—there should be options for everyone. My problem is with label claims that confuse consumers into purchasing products that they think are one thing but really are another. Given the compelling claims made on labels—"safe for mom and baby," "organic, natural girl," and "earth's first"—I was shocked at the amount of harmful chemicals these products contained. It is imperative that we all strive to be part of the solution instead of the problem. I am looking for solutions. To that end, I have included chapters in this book that will teach you how to decipher faulty label claims, and I think you should be able to do pretty well on your own after reading this book.

Because I own a small company and understand the financial hardship of giving away too much product, I was extremely mindful of the burden I might place on a company in conducting this research. For both large and small companies, instead of asking for the product, I offered to pay shipping both ways to borrow the product and look at its ingredients. As an alternative, I told companies that rather than sending the physical product, they could send a list of the ingredients. I want to be clear that I have not tried most of these products. The lists refer to the products' purity, not their efficacy. I would have purchased every single product I researched, but it was simply not feasible. I cannot tell you what levels of the active ingredients they contain. Nor can I tell you how a product feels, smells, or works, factors that vary depending on skin type and individual preference.

These products are not necessarily made the way I would have made them. For instance, some of the mineral makeup contains rice powder, which I consider unnecessary filler—but it won't harm you. To make my "Best" list, a product must be free of all harmful ingredients. For more information on the effectiveness of a product on your body, try asking for samples. My company will send samples of everything; customers who order by mail receive a free sample with each purchase and can request any product to sample with their orders. Additionally, our customers can walk into any Sumbody store and get samples of any product. We are also looking into putting every product in sample sizes so customers can purchase them to test.

Don't forget that just because you see a product from a certain brand does not mean the entire brand is safe. Some companies created one product that is truly natural and ninety-nine products that contain harmful chemicals. I wavered on whether or not to include these companies but decided to follow my principle of searching for solutions. It is important to support the healthy products manufactured by large companies that control a vast market in order to encourage them to create more natural products. In the same way that a sale at Wal-Mart can do more to stimulate the economy than a government tax rebate, so can a large company do more to change the market trend than a small one.

The Learning Curve

Sometimes a little information can go a long way, and sometimes it can go the wrong way. When I first discovered the website Skin Deep, I was so excited by the work it was doing and by the fact that finally there seemed to be an agency taking on the reality of skin care and educating the consumer. I began using it as one of the sources I was relying on it for information regarding ingredients. I was shocked to find that some of the companies I regarded as the forefront of promoting safe and natural products contained ingredients that Skin

Deep rates as hazards. Unwilling to write off these companies without further investigation, I began some in-depth research.

The ingredients in question—such as linalool and limonene—turned out to be naturally occurring components in essential oils. I called the company we order our essential oils from to ask about these compounds. While they are a part of the pure essential oil (not an additive), the company we order from has a machine that analyzes an oil and spits out a data sheet of the percentage of each known allergen within the oil. This company is one of the largest importers and suppliers of essential oils in the country, and I was fortunate to speak not only with its knowledgeable sales reps but with one of its chemists. The data sheets are used primarily by European companies because the labeling laws require known human allergens within essential oils to be declared. Mystery solved. Any product that contains essential oils also contains some of these compounds—even my own. While essential oils are pure and natural, they are also known human allergens. You wouldn't want to soak in pure essential oil or drink it. In my lab we have a ventilation system for handling essential oils. Yes, essential oils contain allergens, but they are not considered caustic or harmful in the concentration they are used in for skin care, nor do they warrant a high hazard rating. Just as some chemical compounds are harmless, some natural ones can pose a threat. I see no problem with essential oils in products, aside from the risk of allergies. (Any time a consumer purchases a product that contains essential oils, he or she should do a batch test by placing a small amount on the inside of their wrist to see if they have a reaction before using.) If I were to rate products using these ingredients as harmful, I would also have to rate every product containing essential oils as harmful, so I am relieved I can include these companies after all.

This experience illustrates how sometimes a little information can rocket us off in the wrong direction. It is extremely important to question everything. If you see a claim, you must ask yourself, "What does it mean?" "How did the producer come to that conclusion?" Do your own research before believing someone else's. Sometimes all we see is one aspect (like the presence of allergens) when we think we're seeing the whole picture. Without the full picture, we can't make a call as to whether or not a certain ingredient or product is (a) what we expect it to be, or (b) safe and natural.

Because of this experience I started to look deeper into the criteria at Skin Deep and look at the studies it cites. Some of them were inconclusive, contained outdated information, and were ambiguous.

During this time I had a customer buy products from Sumbody, go home, read Skin Deep, and absolutely freak out that she was going to die because of what she read. She looked up alcohol on Skin Deep, which received a 10—the most toxic rating—and wanted to return the product for a full refund. When I got a frantic call for my sales associate asking me to call this woman, I already knew what had happened.

When I called the customer back, she turned out to be a lovely woman on a mission to clean out her skin-care products and make healthy choices. She was at the beginning of her learning curve. I explained that while alcohol can cause liver damage and every other problem listed on Skin Deep, these studies focused on the drinking of alcohol over time in larger quantities. I also told her that because over time and in specified quantities alcohol is harmful, I rated alcohol as a potentially harmful ingredient. However, in the quantities that one is exposed to in skin care, I personally find it safe and include it in my products where the alternative chemical I would have to use, which might also cost less, I find to be toxic.

Herein lies the problem. We need proper scientific studies so we have a basis on which to make our choices. A large percentage of the ingredients that I have listed as potentially harmful I feel are harmful, but there is too much conflicting research and inconclusive data to be able to list them as so. This leaves the burden of what to do in your court. My theory is if you just don't know for sure, avoid it. On the other hand, I feel a small percentage of what I have listed as potentially harmful is safe, but again there is conflicting research and enough lingering questions to cause a consumer to be cautious.

Natural herbs and botanicals I have by and large listed as safe if I knew what they were extracted in. However, just because something is from a plant does not mean it is safe or that its safety isn't debatable. As the saying goes, "Too much of a good thing is still too much." Everything has a toxic amount that can harm or kill you, even water.

Even herbs are not without controversy. For some time, the FDA has been trying to regulate and or take herbal supplements off the market due to lack of research.

My next stumble occurred when I did some research into Aubrey Organics. Aubrey was one of the first companies to make natural products, and when I began purchasing my own products at a young age, it was one of my first picks. Its products are relatively inexpensive and readily available, and I wanted to be able to promote something in this book that everyone could find. I hoped to tout Aubrey as the forefront of the industry. When I inspected its labels, everything looked great except the presence of a "coconut fatty acid cream base" in some products and "coconut oil-corn oil soap" in others. I called the company. The customer-service representative with whom I spoke did not know what was in the corn and coconut base. She transferred me to someone who she said would know the answer. She didn't. So I asked for the proper ingredient declaration or Latin for the base, but she didn't know that either. Corn oil and coconut oil sound great, but they do not lather, which is what the base is supposed to do. Knowing there was something missing, I asked to speak with the chemist, who was unavailable and has not yet e-mailed me a response at the time of this book's printing.

This is one of the trickiest situations for a consumer, because even if you've read the label and called the company, you might still be fooled. The average consumer should not have to be able to analyze the ingredients and determine that the product is missing a lathering agent and therefore there must be something else in it. "Coconut oil-corn oil soap" *sounds* safe. This is where you have to be especially vigilant because companies are clever. Lumping ingredients into something that sounds harmless, like a base or a mix, is dangerous because you don't know what is in that base, even if the label says it is coconut and corn. How are they kept together? What form are they in? Are they extracted in a third substance? Do they contain additives? All of these are questions you must ask yourself. Before you trust a company's "all-natural base," be sure you know exactly what is in it—every single ingredient. Additionally, you should never trust something just because the label claims it is derived from coconut or any other natural substance. One of the most widely acknowledged toxic ingredients on the market right now is dioxane, which is derived from coconut. But by the time it becomes dioxane, it is a completely new substance; the fact that it once was a part of a coconut is meaningless in determining its safety. I am not saying that Aubrey is not natural or is trying to deceive us, but since I was unable to obtain a straight answer about some questionable ingredient declarations, I cannot verify that these products are safe. If you want to consider Aubrey as an option, do your own research and make sure you are satisfied with the answers. It is up to you to decide.

Who Owns Whom?

Don't let the brand name fool you. Even if you have come to love, believe, and trust in the story and image of a brand, take a second look. Read each and every label carefully. Green personal care is big business. It means big money for major companies. They buy up and market the green magic that smaller brands have created. In most cases the "natural" component of the company they are buying is just a sales tool invented to get consumer dollars. They are buying a tale, a story that the brand has created, and an image that consumers have come to trust. In other cases the company might have been natural and green, but once the larger companies get involved things change. If it becomes profitable to them to keep these green brands green, they will. This is where the consumer comes in. The more you demand, the more educated you become, the cleaner and better options you will have.

The following are examples of some of the most recent buyouts of some of the best-known "natural" brands:

- ◇ Burt's Bees was purchased by Clorox for $913 million.
- ◇ Aveda was purchased by Estée Lauder for $300 million.
- ◇ Tom's of Maine was purchased by Colgate-Palmolive for $100 million.
- ◇ The Body Shop was purchased by L'Oréal for $1.4 billion.

Natural is not small business anymore. This makes it imperative that we as consumers become more vigilant. We need to understand just what is in our products, so we can make choices we believe in, not choices we are sold.

Criteria for Alternative Options

In the chapters to come, I'll be giving you my recommendations for natural alternatives to conventional products. When using these lists, keep my criteria in mind. The products I've chosen are those with the most natural ingredients and the least harmful synthetic ones. This is not a statement about the overall company, and things can change fast in this industry. For example, Burt's Bee's was bought out twice, most recently by Clorox. In this climate of constant mergers and acquisitions, there's no way to predict which company will own which at any given time, and ownership changes can lead to change in a product's formula, so please continue to read labels.

Also, there are some products listed that are clean and natural, but *everything* else the company makes is loaded with chemicals. So do not assume that if a company has one product listed, everything it makes is good.

Additionally, I either denote specific flavors/scents (such as when a company has salt scrubs in a variety of scents), which implies the flavors/scents not listed include fragrance, or I list a product without specifying flavors/scents. In the latter case, it means that all of the flavors/scents were OK at the time I checked. Companies are constantly changing flavors/scents and creating new ones, so while they were all OK when I checked them, I do not feel comfortable making a blanket statement about things that might change a week after this book is published.

These lists provide you with a wide range of products to choose from. Still, they are not the only ones that fit into these categories. I would love to be able to review every natural product available, but that would be impossible. I simply could not find them all. If you know of products that should be included, I would like to hear about them. I love to spread the word on companies making products using little or no chemicals.

In the following chapters, you will find product categories, followed by a list of alternative products ranked "Good," "Better," or

"Best" in terms of exposure to harmful chemicals. When creating the criteria for these lists, the first thing I did was take my own advice. I sat down and made a list of the top ten or so chemicals I absolutely would not allow on my skin. From there, it got tricky. I had to sift through questions about ingredients that posed a lesser threat, as well as harmful ingredients that appear in small amounts. What if the product contains all natural ingredients except for one hazardous one? What are the extracts extracted in? My inability to plot out exact criteria illustrates the core of the issue with the beauty industry and the reason I am writing this book. The line between natural and synthetic blurs more each day, and the information out there can be manipulated to support any argument. Further problems bubbled up as I considered a criterion that could span the multitude of products I cover; I had to make compromises.

Consider shampoo. There really is no completely natural lathering agent except for pure Castile soap, which is made from natural vegetable oils—traditionally pure olive oil—and sodium carbonate (lye, which is not present in the finished soap). If this were the end of the story, it would be simple—I would place all shampoos with a Castile soap base in the "Best" category and move on. Unfortunately, it isn't this simple. While it has the lather, Castile soap is thin and watery, with none of the gel consistency we expect and love from our shampoos. Most people don't like the way it makes their hair feel. The point of the "Good," "Better," "Best" lists is to provide consumers with options for natural products that they can switch to without losing any, or many, of the characteristics they expect from their more harmful product. I had to include shampoo that fit this standard as well as a standard of health, and this is where I was forced to compromise. Some of the shampoos I have included contain ingredients that I would not let near a face scrub or cleanser, but they were the best available.

I took into consideration everything from how many synthetic ingredients were in a product and whether or not any of them were toxic to the level of toxicity, backed by data from sources including medical dictionaries, chemical companies, material safety data sheets (MSDSs), poison control centers, the Skin Deep website, and information from other watchdog groups and nonprofit organizations. I dissected every product from many angles. I am a purist who believes that if we would not eat an ingredient, we should not slather it on our bodies, so I asked myself, "Would you eat a teaspoon of this chemical? Would you eat an eighth of a teaspoon?" and "Would I rub this on my skin if it were not suspended in other ingredients?" If I answered no, I was again faced with the need to compromise some of my personal standards to create an accessible list. The "Alternative Options" lists allow people to choose their own level of comfort rather than having to adhere to mine. I could easily do a chemical-free makeover with 100 percent healthy and effective products, but that isn't the point of this list—I want to give people options for all budgets and ranges of accessibility.

While I did include a certain number of synthetic ingredients, I kept coming back to the question of whether or not I would rub it on my skin or whether I could eat it if I had to. I ploughed through MSDSs and spoke with several chemists from leading chemical companies. While most of them are pro-chemical, particularly if you say, "I'm going to have OSHA out at my site and I want to make sure I abide by all the industry regulations," they can provide you with much good information. If an employee has a rash, they'll give you thorough instructions on what to do. Hearing the disposal regulations for some of these chemicals was a huge eye-opener for me—I could rub a certain chemical all over my body, but I could not let a drop spill onto the earth? I delved into all of the resources available to me as a consumer, businesswoman, and formulator and fused all of them together to form a shifting, all-encompassing criterion. If someone told me a company was all natural and it was not on the Internet, I would call the company, and if it would not release its ingredients over the phone, I would find a local retailer and go to the store and physically copy down the ingredients on the container so I could research them myself. If I was unable to find a store where the products were sold, I would go to even greater extremes. I don't think anyone should have to go to these lengths in order to determine what is in his or her body-care products.

Consider a company called Pomega5, for example. I saw a pamphlet for its products and wanted to investigate further. First I searched the Internet, but the products' ingredients were not listed. Luckily, there was a phone number on the contact page, which I promptly called. I was greeted by an answering service, and the woman I spoke with told me I could not speak directly with a representative from Pomega5, but I could leave a message and someone would get back to me. This is the point where, if I were only looking for products as a consumer, I would have given up and found a different product. I pressed on because these products are carried in Whole Foods, which is a relatively accessible store for most people, albeit a bit pricey. I dug and dug for days and finally unearthed enough information about the company to include several products in the "Good," "Better," "Best" list. In all fairness, they did list an e-mail address on the contact page in addition to a phone number. This experience reinforced the importance of companies displaying their ingredient decks online. Consumers should not have to wait a week or longer to find out what is in a product they are interested in purchasing. Additionally, if companies are required to list the ingredients on the back of each product, why should they be able to circumvent this by selling on the Internet? Yes, the ingredients may be listed once you receive the product, but consumers should have access to the full ingredient list at the point of purchase, whether at their local drug store or from an online vendor.

In devising my own criteria, I took a look at what else is out there. During the course of writing this book, I became even better acquainted with the website Skin Deep, operated by the Environmental Working Group. I had never consulted the website when formulating my own products because I already have a standard for ingredients I will use, but a chemist I have worked with for years told me that he will not formulate products for a natural company without consulting Skin Deep on each ingredient. This is not because he thinks Skin Deep is correct, but because the public trusts it as the watchdog for ingredients, and if an ingredient is rated high on Skin Deep, even if he doesn't think it is harmful, he won't formulate with it because he doesn't want to risk the company's ability to market its product.

Skin Deep rates products as well as ingredients. One day I sat down and tried to figure out its criteria, but I couldn't. One of the products contained an ingredient with a rating of six, and yet the product had an overall rating of three. While I am assuming this is because it was added in a small quantity, or it was the only harmful ingredient, or relative to the other products on the market it was an overall three, I cannot say for sure. The closest I could find to a criterion was an overall explanation, but this did not cover the rhyme or reason for rating specific products. When I called the California branch of Skin Deep, the person I spoke to could not answer my question but did say I could set up an interview with the founder of Skin Deep in Washing, Delaware, who could probably answer that question. I would love to meet with her not only for an answer to that question but also for the opportunity to pick the brain behind one of the largest efforts to rate the safety of cosmetic ingredients and make that information accessible to the public. Unfortunately, I could not schedule an interview before the publication date for this book. My assumption is that Skin Deep devised its criteria much the way I've devised mine, considering the product on its own but also in relation to other products on the market; the level of potentially toxic substances; the number of synthetic ingredients; and the type of base they are suspended in.

The "Alternative Options" lists are truly a labor of love, and anyone is welcome to e-mail me with questions about my selections; I'll do my best to explain my reasoning.

One company that spells out its criterion is Lush. Each of its products is color-coded to indicate a natural product or a product made with safe synthetics. This allows consumers to choose their level of comfort and make purchases accordingly. Under "safe synthetics," it lists propylene glycol, sodium lauryl sulfate, and parabens—ingredients I would consider anything but safe. Still, the disclosure is a step in the right direction. At least it isn't claiming these ingredients are "all natural." But by now you know not to trust everything you read. Just because the producer considers it a safe synthetic does not mean you will—never stop reading labels! This is a beginning, and I would love to hear from other companies that are posting similar standards. Of course, there is a big difference between good ingredients and efficacy, texture, and absorption—a product can be all-natural without working, but that doesn't mean it can't be both natural *and* effective. The dialogue about questioning and inspecting labels and searching for truly natural products has begun, and I hope my next book will contain lists that are bigger and better, until consumers can finally choose from an encyclopedia of "Best" products in the same way that we can now grab chemical-filled ones off any shelf.

I hope the readers of this book will fill my e-mail box with the names of truly natural companies that I have missed. I hope companies will willingly provide samples or ingredient lists, so I do not have to hunt them down. I hope that as consumers demand more, we will see things change more rapidly in the future. I hope we will come to expect all "natural"-labeled personal-care products and companies to do the following:

⬧ have customer service that responds to the concerns of the buyer and will answer questions
⬧ have company criteria that are spelled out and adhered to
⬧ disclose all ingredients both on labels and websites
⬧ have no hidden ingredients
⬧ adopt product-development practices that take both the consumer's health and that of the planet into account
⬧ use cutting-edge natural ingredients that have beneficial results
⬧ refuse to use products that have been tested on animals
⬧ take into account the impact on the planet of their ingredients, manufacture, packaging, and sourcing
⬧ make products of food-grade quality
⬧ market honestly and openly
⬧ educate consumers so they can make choices they believe in
⬧ be subject to standards in the beauty industry that are comparable with those in the food industry.

The following are some quick tips to remember when looking at products on the "Good," "Better," "Best" lists:

1. I have not tried the products. I am vouching for their purity, not their efficacy.

2. Although an ingredient may be harmless, I cannot say that they are ingredients I believe are effective for what they are being used for, are necessarily beneficial for your skin, or exist in levels that will work.

3. I cannot vouch for the companies that produce them.

4. Please remember that just because you see a product from a company listed, that does not mean that everything or anything else they make is clean, safe, or chemical-free.

Remember that all skin is different. What works for one person may not work for someone else.

These simple tips will make it possible for you to evaluate the products in the chapters that follow, so you can safely see if they fit into your criteria for a product you feel comfortable using. They are also a reminder to test the product's efficacy for yourself. Being safe and effective are two very different things.

The following chapters will show you what an average body-care product is made of, why certain ingredients are harmful, and how you can reap the benefits you want without compromising your health or budget. Keep in mind that while some of the conventional products I've listed contain beneficial ingredients like avocado oil or apricot oil, that doesn't make the product healthy or safe. Most of these good ingredients are not used in amounts large enough to qualify them as active ingredients, and on the chance that one is, the effect may be mitigated by the abundance of synthetic chemicals accompanying it.

Every label has a 1 percent line, which means that after a certain point, ingredients are used in quantities of 1 percent or less. So while avocado oil sounds enticing, there might be no more than two drops in every gallon of product. If a cake looked delicious and claimed vitamins and health benefits but was made of petroleum products, you wouldn't eat it; the same is true for bath products.

Chapter 7

Bath Salts, Teas, Oils, Melts, Bombs/Fizzies/Fizzers, Confetti/Caviar

I thought a lot about whether or not to include my own products on the "Good," "Better," and "Best" lists because I didn't want doing so to discredit my knowledge and passion for healthy beauty products by making readers think I wrote this book simply to promote my brand. On the other hand, I feel as though leaving my products out would beg the question as to why, with all this knowledge, I have not managed to formulate safe and healthy products. Therefore, I feel the presence of Sumbody products on these lists proves my ability to "walk the walk." That said, I was scrupulous about making sure my products held up to the same standards I applied to the other products on these lists, and the few products of mine that fell short were not included.

Having the spa experience at home has become a huge hit with consumers. Not everyone has the time or money to visit a spa regularly. It is much more cost-effective for people to carve out time for a relaxing bath or add a spa treatment to their shower. The products used for these pleasant, relaxing, and healthful spa experiences form an important category in the personal-care industry. They are all about pampering, relaxing, taking time for yourself, and feeling good. In the fast-paced, crazy world we live in, they help us to unwind, let go, and reconnect with ourselves. They allow us to take a moment to pamper ourselves.

When you soak in a tub or apply a product in the shower, your pores absorb more because they are open as a result of the heat. And when you take a bath, you tend to spend a little more time than you do when you shower. The soaking allows more of the ingredients in the products to be absorbed.

Most products in this category need only very basic ingredients to be effective, so there is an abundance of truly natural products available.

Bath Salts

Bath salts are one of the most popular types of products in this category. These rejuvenating salts are used for everything from reducing muscle tension to detoxification to simple relaxation. Each salt claims a unique property. The common unnecessary ingredients to look for in bath salts are fragrance, surfactants (lathering agents), artificial colors, preservatives, and petroleum products. Bath salts can be produced without any of these ingredients. Look for products that do not foam or lather and that contain pure sea salts, essential oils, natural oils such as avocado or sunflower, and mica for color. Since salt is a natural preservative, without water present in the product, there is no need for additional preservatives. To prevent contamination after you have opened a jar of bath salts, keep hands, water, and anything such as food or dirt from entering the jar. Purchase airtight jars or bags that allow you to pour a desired amount of salts directly into the tub and reseal. Even if you choose to scoop, or keep your salts in an open dish by your tub, it is highly unlikely that they will become contaminated. The salt in your kitchen is unpreserved. We cook with it, keep it for long periods, and never worry about handling, touching, or eating it.

When choosing bath salts, look for companies that use sea salt. Sea salt is harvested from evaporated seawater. This seawater has additional minerals that are beneficial to the skin, relax muscle tension, and have other positive attributes, such as detoxification, that are beneficial for use in skin care. Sea salt is not limited to only sodium and chloride that make up the traditional salt molecule.

Table salt lacks the additional minerals found in sea salt and can contain additives such as the anticaking agent silicon dioxide, the primary ingredient in sand and iodine.

Here is an ingredient list for a bath salt that illustrates things to avoid:

- magnesium sulfate
- potassium alum
- sodium cocoyl isethionate
- cocamidopropyl betaine
- mineral oil
- phenoxyethanol
- fragrance

May contain:
- FD&C Yellow 5, Blue 1, D&C Red 33

(Notice there is not even any real sea salt which is the primary active ingredient in bath salts. Some of the benefits of sea salt are they detoxify, relax, release muscle tension, and soften skin.)

Contrast this with an ingredient list for a bath salt containing helpful ingredients to look for:

- solar evaporated sea salt
- pure essential oil blend

Alternative Options for Least Amount of Added Toxins—Bath Salts

GOOD

1. Hugo Natural Botanical Apothecary Effervescent Bath Salts: French Lavender, Geranium

BETTER

1. Sumbody Sel de Mer Bath Salts

BEST

1. EO Bath Salts: Rose Geranium and Citrus
2. Jasco Organics Sea Salts
3. Back Porch Soap Company Sea Salt Soak for Tub & Jacuzzi
4. Best Bath Store Dead Sea Salts
5. Lunaroma Bath Salts
6. Lunaroma Caribbean Herbal Bath Salts
7. Wild Woozle Soap Company After Yoga Bath Soak
8. Sumbody Let My Muscles Go Bath Salts
9. Sumbody Mustard Bath Salts
10. Sumbody Stress Relief Bath Salts

> **TIP**
> Mix pure sea salt and Epsom salts (available at any drugstore) with essential oils. The label should read "pure sea salt" (make sure not to use table salt; see above). To find essential oils, look at your local drug or health-food store or shop online. Make sure they are called pure essential oils—not essence or fragrance.

Bath Teas

Bath teas can be loose or packaged in large tea bags. They infuse bathwater with herbs, flowers, or botanicals and can provide soothing, energy, or skin-repair benefits. They are a good alternative for people who find bath salts drying. The common unnecessary ingredients to look for in bath teas are the same as those in bath salts: fragrance, artificial colors, preservatives, and petroleum products. Look for teas that contain essential oils and pure oils, such as apricot or sunflower, and that do not foam or lather. Just like drinking teas, bath teas do not need preservatives.

Here is an ingredient list for a bath tea that illustrates things to avoid:

- lavender (*Lavandula angustifolia*) petals
- rose petals (*Rosa canina*)
- black tea (*Camellia sinensis*)
- phenoxyethanol
- fragrance
- D&C Violet 2

Contrast this with an ingredient list for a bath tea containing helpful ingredients to look for:

- calendula (*Calendula officinalis*) petals
- chamomile (*Matricaria recutita*) flower
- comfrey (*Symphytum officinale*) leaf
- juniper berry (*Juniperus communis*)
- oats (*Avena sativa*)
- rosemary (*Rosmarinus officinalus*) leaf
- sage (*Salvia officinalis*) leaf
- orrisroot (*Iris germanica*)
- bergamot (*Monarda didyma*) oil

Alternative Options for Least Amount of Added Toxins— Bath Teas

I did the math several times over, and if you buy herbal tea and use two to three bags in your bath, it is cheaper than most bath teas. The only difference is marketing, and sometimes the bath teas contain essential oils.

Use any brand of drinking tea, including the following:

- peppermint for energy
- rose-hip, green, black, or white for skin repair
- cold-care teas when you're coming down with a cold
- rooibos or honeybush for relaxing

If you want to purchase one premade tea:

| BEST

1. Sumbody Geranium Detox Bath Tea

2. Delights of the Earth Bath Tea: Relaxing, Soothing, Therapeutic

> **TIP** Place your regular loose drinking tea in a reusable muslin bag and add two drops of essential oils to your bath for a relaxing home-spa treatment.

Bath Oils and Melts

Bath oils and melts are a great way to enjoy aromatherapy and moisturize your skin. I have put them in one category since their benefits are the same. The difference is that bath oil is in a liquid form and a melt is solid. Melts are made in molds and can be found in a variety of appealing shapes and sizes. Moisturizing in the tub or shower provides a much deeper penetration and is a great way to rehydrate. There are two basic reasons for this: The warm water opens your pores, allowing for better absorption; and since you lose most of your moisture in the first five minutes after you're out of the shower/bath, moisturizing in the shower/bath can help prevent that loss. Please remember that these products make surfaces slippery, so use caution when getting into and out of the bath or shower.

The common unnecessary ingredients to look for in bath oils and melts are cheap filler oils made from petroleum, or other toxic bases, fragrance, artificial colors, preservatives, extracts, and chemicals that allow the oil to mix with water so that it is suspended in the bath as opposed to floating on top. Look for bath oils made using pure food-grade oils, such as avocado, grape seed, or almond, as well as pure essential oils and plant extracts that are extracted in pure oil.

Here is an ingredient list for a bath melt that illustrates things to avoid:

- cocoa (*Theobroma cacao*) butter
- laureth-4
- almond (*Prunus amygdalus*) oil
- lavender (*Lavandula angustifolia*) oil
- jasmine (*Jasminum officinale*) flower
- geraniol

- limonene
- linalool
- perfume

Contrast this with an ingredient list for a bath melt containing helpful ingredients to look for:*

- cocoa (*Theobroma cacao*) butter
- extracts of motherwort (*Leonurus cardiaca*)
- gotu kola (*Centella asiatica*)
- calendula (*Calendula officinalis*) petals
- essential oil blend

* Note that this product is marketed as cocoa butter, not as a bath melt.

Alternative Options for Least Amount of Added Toxins— Bath Oils and Melts

| BEST

1. See "Body Oils" on pages 107–109. You can eliminate the purchase of an additional product and use your body oil in the bath. Also, this way you will go through the one product faster and it will be fresher.
2. Sumbody Bath Melt
3. Chagrin Valley Soap and Craft Company Cocoa Butter Bath Melt

TIP Mix the olive, avocado, safflower, or grape seed oil you use for cooking with two drops of essential oil, and add to your bath.

Bath Bombs/Fizzies/Fizzers

Bath bombs come in many shapes and sizes, with many different names, such as fizzies and fizzers, but they all do the same thing. They release effervescence and claim a variety of mood-altering and medicinal properties. Although they fizz instead of foaming or creating bubbles, many people use them as a safe alternative to conventional bubble baths. These are popular with children and teenagers as well as adults. Whenever you bathe in something (sit for extended periods in your bath absorbing it), it is extremely important to know what you're soaking in. These products, like those you don't wash off, are the ones the skin is most exposed to. Aside from the fact that synthetic ingredients can be cheaper, there is no reason to use any harmful ingredients in a bath bomb. In most cases, you can find natural ones at the same price as the artificial ones. The common unnecessary ingredients to look for in bath bombs are fragrance, artificial colors, preservatives, and petroleum products, chemicals that are used as cheap fillers and foaming agents. Some of the beneficial ingredients you should look for in a bath bomb are pure oils, butters, and pure essential oils.

Here is the ingredient list for a fizzer that illustrates things to avoid:

- sodium bicarbonate
- citric acid
- perfume
- mineral oil
- aqua (water)
- hydroxyisohexyl 3-cyclohexene
- carboxaldehyde
- FD&C Yellow 5
- FD&C Blue 1
- mica
- titanium dioxide
- geraniol
- farnesol
- limonene
- linalool
- D&C Violet 2

Contrast this with an ingredient list for a fizzer containing helpful ingredients to look for:

- sodium bicarbonate
- citric acid
- witch hazel (*Hamamelis virginiana*)
- shea (*Butyrospermum parkii*) butter
- orange peel (*Citrus aurantium*)
- orange (*Citrus sinensis*) essential oil
- grapefruit (*Citrus paradisi*) essential oil
- lemon (*Citrus medica limonum*) essential oil
- lime (*Citrus aurantifolia*) essential oil

Alternative Options for Least Amount of Added Toxins— Bath Bombs/Fizzies/Fizzers

GOOD

1. Wild Woozle Soap Company Fizzy Hydrotherapy Bath Powder: You're the Bomb

2. Lush Bath Bomb: Honey Lumps, Retro Lush, Tisty Tosty

3. Shebas Secrets: Bath Bomb Fizzies, Dirty Bombs, and Busy Bee Bombs

BETTER

1. Sumbody Bath Fizzer: Get Lei'd, Coconut & Cream

BEST

1. Best Bath Store Dead Sea Bath Bomb

2. Best Bath Store Bath Bomb: Lavender, Detox, Eucalyptus, Lemon Poppy, Lemon Lime, Orange, Orange Ylang Ylang, Rose, Rose Heart. (Note that online several flavors of this product look dyed, but no dye is listed except beet powder. I have used beet powder many times to dye these products and it does not look like that. I am giving the company the benefit of doubt and assuming that they used Photoshop to alter the color.)

3. Sumbody Bath Fizzer: Tsunami, California Sunshine, Lavender Splash, Lavender Dream, Mustard Detox, Milky Rich

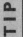 **TIP** Use a bath bomb/fizzer with moisturizer; with your pores open, you'll get the fullest benefit from moisturizing while you relax in the tub.

Bath Confetti/Caviar

Bath confetti/caviars are soaks that are largely used for scent and color. They do not have beneficial properties and are what I consider novelty or "for fun" products. There are many brands that are targeted to children and teens. The bright, fake colors and bold fragrance and festive packaging stand out to the under-eighteen market. They are common in kits and gift sets, and tend to bubble. I have not been able to find natural alternatives.

Here is an ingredient list for a bath confetti that illustrates things to avoid:

- potato (*Solanum tuberosum*)
- polyvinyl alcohol
- sodium lauryl sulfate
- cocamidopropyl betaine
- glycerin
- cocamide MEA
- water
- perfume
- methylparaben
- allantoin
- butylated hydroxytoluene (BHT)

May contain:
- D&C Red 33, FD&C Yellow 5, FD&C Blue 1, FD&C Red 40

Here is an ingredient list for a bath caviar that illustrates things to avoid:

- urea
- VP/VA copolymer
- mica
- fragrance
- benzophenone-2

May contain:
- FD&C Yellow 5, FD&C Blue 1, D&C Red 33, FD&C Yellow 6

Alternative Options for Least Amount of Added Toxins— Bath Confetti/Caviar

I could not find any products in this category that could even be listed as "Good." I'm sure they exist, and I'd love to hear about them, but I don't have any to recommend. Since these products are just for fun and provide no benefit, I suggest using bath products that are not only fun but also provide benefits. There are plenty of options within the overall product list.

Chapter 8

Lotions, Lotion Bars, Body Butters, and Oils

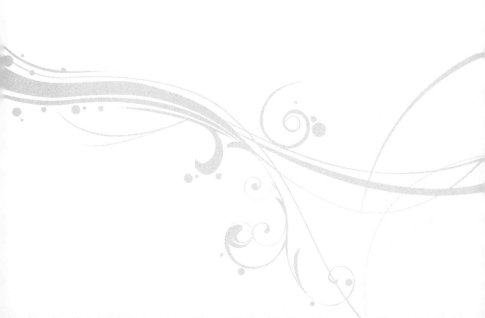

Body moisturizers are a great place to make a change. There are a few different categories in personal care: things we soak in, things we wash off, and things we leave on. The products we leave on allow for the most absorption of the ingredients. Products we soak in are the next concern, and ones we and wash off are the least concerning. Both because we leave lotions on and because of the amount of surface they cover (from neck to toe), it is very important to find one you like that is within your comfort range when it comes to chemical exposure.

Most commercial moisturizers are made to feel good when going on but do nothing to reduce dryness. In fact, most are made with chemicals that actually dry your skin. A good moisturizer should replenish your body's natural oils, as well as trap its existing moisture. A moisturizer can be any lotion, oil, body butter, or bar that seals the moisture in so that your skin cannot dehydrate as easily or quickly. The addition of rich hydrating ingredients that moisturize or heal dry skin is a bonus.

Because dry skin is both uncomfortable and (to some) unsightly, the cosmetic industry has made a fortune selling us skin savers in a jar. Companies advertise herbs and extracts for antiwrinkle properties, and milk and oats for added moisturizing effects. They promise us everything from "smooth-as-silk" skin to skin that "feels like a baby's." The quest for relief and attractive skin leads the consumer on a bottle-by-bottle search for the perfect moisturizing miracle. It is this very search that has driven both the increased sales of body moisturizers and the increase in dry skin.

Body moisturizers have become significantly more popular with the increase in dry skin. Ironically it is the application of these products that is one of the contributors to this increase. If you look at the ingredient list for 99 percent of all body lotions, you will find petroleum-based ingredients, alcohol, fragrance, and other chemicals, such as "-cones" (for more on -cones see the discussions on pages 155 and

204) and preservatives. Although some of these ingredients make the product feel better when you apply it, they ultimately damage and dry out your skin. So the more lotion you use to combat your dry skin, the dryer it will become and the more you will "need." The more you "soak" in luxurious bubble bath and lather with conventional soap, the more problems you create by further drying out your skin.

Along with the increase of dry skin, we are seeing an increase in allergies and sensitivities to lotions. Skin is being overexposed to harmful ingredients through the addition of new and more chemicals to body lotions. With so much contact, with so many chemicals and chemical combinations, it is no wonder more and more people are having sensitivity issues. This exposure can cause havoc for skin, leading to symptoms such as redness, irritation, inching, rashes, and a slew of other skin-care issues.

Besides being uncomfortable, if left untreated, dry skin can lead to dermatitis—an inflammation of the skin—swelling, and infection. Dry skin is also more prone to sensitivity.

The best way to reduce and heal dry skin is to decrease the underlying causes while adopting habits that will help prevent it. You will use less lotion, save money, and help your skin simply by changing the current products you are using and adding some dry-skin prevention tricks to your regimen.

The following are some additional causes for dry skin to watch out for:

- dry climates
- overchlorinated tap water, as well as other tap- and well-water elements (such as softeners that cause drying)
- exposure to sun, wind, cold, and smog
- exposure to chemicals
- excess bathing and exposure to water
- chlorinated pools or hot tubs
- harsh body soap/laundry soap
- medications
- irritating clothing

Lotions/Creams

Basic lotion is an emulsion of oil in water. In order to get the oil and water to mix, an emulsifier is required. However, with today's technology, chemists can make a lotion without using any real oils at all. Some lotions merely consist of a synthetic chemical smorgasbord. Body lotions are very similar to face creams in how they are made and how they work. Lotions made with chemicals tend to mask underlying issues and give a "feel factor" that is virtually impossible to re-create naturally. When you apply them, your skin feels wonderful to the touch. Don't always believe what you feel. These lotions can contain "-cones," alcohol, fragrance, and other ingredients that not only dry out your skin but also accelerate the aging process. Natural lotions may not give the same "ahh" effect, but over time they will make your skin look and feel better. The oils and butters in these lotions help trap moisture in your skin to prevent dehydration and replenish lost moisture. In the long run you will notice your skin looking naturally awesome, even though you are using less product.

Look for lotions that are rich in butters and oils such as shea butter, almond oil, and avocado oil. Reduce the amount of chemicals you are applying by simply choosing products with fewer synthetic chemicals. Everyone is different, so choose what you like the feel of, but generally speaking, from the neck down your skin needs the richer butters for the right kind of moisture.

Here is an ingredient list for a body lotion that illustrates things to avoid:

- water
- glycerin
- caprylic/capric triglyceride
- babassu (*Orbignya oleifera*) oil
- sweet almond (*Prunus amygdalus dulcis*) oil
- fragrance
- dimethicone
- methyl glucose sesquistearate
- PEG-20 methyl glucose sesquistearate
- phenoxyethanol
- shea (*Butyrospermum parkii*) butter
- carbomer

- sodium hydroxide
- methylparaben
- geraniol
- alpha-isomethyl ionone
- lily of the valley (*Convallaria majalis*) bulb/root extract
- disodium EDTA
- butylparaben
- ethylparaben
- citronellal
- isobutylparaben
- propylparaben

Contrast this with an ingredient list for a body lotion containing healthful ingredients to look for:

- purified water
- organic lavender (*Lavandula angustifolia*) hydrosol
- vegetable emulsifying wax NF
- organic sunflower (*Helianthus annuus*) oil
- organic unrefined beeswax (*Cera alba*)
- wild-crafted Brazil nut (*Bertholletia excelsa*) oil
- wild-crafted andiroba (*Carapa guianensis*) oil
- lavender (*Lavandula angustifolia*) essential oil
- petitgrain (*Citrus aurantium*) essential oil
- ylang-ylang (*Cananga odorata*) essential oil
- patchouli (*Pogostemon cablin*) essential oil
- vegetable-derived stearic acid
- vitamins A, C , and E
- extracts of oregano (*Origanum vulgare*), thyme (*Thymus vulgaris*), cinnamon (*Cinnamomum zeylanicum*), rosemary (*Rosmarinus officinalis*), lavender (*Lavender angustifolia*), goldenseal (*Hydrastis canadensis*), and neem (*Melia azadirachta*) extracted in safflower (*Carthamus tinctorius*) oil

Alternative Options for Least Amount of Added Toxins— Lotions/Creams

GOOD

1. Botanical Skin Works Shea Butter Face & Body Lotion
2. Botanical Skin Works Vitamin E Cream

3. Wild Woozle Soap Company Ginger Marmalade Firming Body Lotion

| BETTER

1. Hugo Natural Botanical Apothecary All Over Lotion: French Lavender, Spearmint

| BEST

1. Nature's Gate Rainwater Organics Lotion with Acai Oil
2. Dr. Hauschka Quince Body Moisturizer
3. Uhma Nagri Shower Lotion: Rose
4. Uhma Nagri All Natural Body Cream: Copacabana Mango
5. Uhma Nagri Copacabana All Natural Body Lotion: Mango
6. Badger Bali Balm
7. Suki Velvet Moisturizing Cream
8. In Fiore Body Balm
9. Ciao Bella Replenishing Body Lotion
10. Hugo Natural Botanical Apothecary Cucumber & Geranium Body Butter
11. Hugo French Lavender Body Butter
12. Sumbody Silk Amino Body Lotion
13. Sumbody Goat Milk Body Cream
14. Sumbody Butter Me Up Body Butter

Lotion Bars

This form of moisturizer has become popular and widely available over the last fifteen years, although I imagine there was a historic version, given the availability of butters and ease of production. The first lotion bar I ever saw was from a company called Lush, and I loved the concept immediately. There is no water, making preservation easier, no need to emulsify, and reduced packaging, and these moisturizers can be made from a variety of luscious skin-loving butters. If you like the feel and texture of a bar lotion, you won't have a hard time finding one that is chemical-free. There is no reason to settle for a bar with chemical additives. However, look out for fragrance, parabens, and other unnecessary additives. Look for bars with pure essential oils, true butters, and no artificial colorants. The conventional bar listed below appears on the surface to be not that bad. I listed it because it illustrates a key problem. It lists both fresh lemon and fresh mango. Although they are both good for your skin, when they are used in a product, they require preservation. If you leave a fresh lemon or mango open outside of the refrigerator, it will go bad. What is preserving these ingredients in this bar? If you were to use only butters and oils, it would be stable. Consider how long an open bottle of oil can last in your kitchen. Additionally, with fresh lemon being the second ingredient and ingredients being listed in order of amount from most to least, everything after cocoa butter must be present in tiny amounts. How could the product be a bar if it were half fresh lemon? Thus, this is really a bar of cocoa butter with a few other ingredients added in small amounts.

Here is an ingredient list for a lotion bar that illustrates things to avoid:

- fair-trade cocoa (*Theobroma cacao*) butter
- fresh lemon (*Citrus limon*)
- shea (*Butyrospermum parkii*) butter
- fresh mango (*Mangifera indica*)
- horsetail (*Equisetum arvense*)
- cleavers (*Galium aparine*)
- vanilla pod (*Vanilla planifolia*) infusion
- lanolin
- perfume
- hydrogenated palm (*Elaeis guineensis*) kernel oil
- coconut (*Cocos nucifera*) butter
- beeswax (*Cera alba*)
- wheat-germ (*Triticum vulgare*) oil
- soybean (*Glycine soja*) oil
- shea (*Butyrospermum parkii*) butter
- cardamom (*Elettaria cardamomum*) oil
- vanilla absolute (*Vanilla planifolia*)
- neroli (*Citrus amara*) oil
- lavender (*Lavandula hybrida*) oil

- paprika (*Capsicum frutescens*) extract
- citral
- geraniol
- limonene
- linalool
- coumarin
- hydroxycitronellal

Contrast this with an ingredient list of a lotion bar containing helpful ingredients to look for:

- cocoa (*Theobroma cacao*) butter
- shea (*Butyrospermum parkii*) butter
- beeswax (*Cera alba*)
- lavender (*Lavandula angustifolia*) essential oil

Alternative Options for Least Amount of Added Toxins— Lotion Bars

GOOD

1. Lush After 8:30 Massage Bar (Retro Lush)

BETTER

2. Sumbody Palm It: Sex on the Beach

BEST

1. Lush Each Peach Massage Bar
2. Wild Woozle Soap Company Meditation Massage Bar
3. Sumbody Palm It: Love, Relaxation, Joy
4. Chagrin Valley Soap and Craft Company Three Butter Lotion Bar
5. Chagrin Valley Soap and Craft Company Hemp Mango Mint Lotion Bar

Body Butters

Body butters are usually very thick lotions, sometimes thicker than a cream, with butters in the ingredient list. Depending on the amount of butters used, they can be extra rich and moisturizing. In nature, there are very few real butters. Real butters, such as sal, shea, mowrah, murumuru, cocoa, cupuaçu, and mango, come from a specific natural source, with no added ingredients, and they can sometimes be found packaged as body butters. To the best of my knowledge, these are the only real butters. Avocado, olive, almond, and aloe butter are not naturally occurring butters. They are a combination of the oil (or in the case of aloe, the juice) stearic acid to make a "butter." Look for these in your body butter ingredients lists. You will pay more for the butter, but it is no different from the oil and has no additional moisturizing properties. In fact, it is cheaper for the company to add the stearic acid than it is to leave the oil pure.

Another form of body butter is a blend of butter or butters with an oil to give a smoother texture. These can be made like a lotion bar and sold in a pot. Like lotion bars, they require less preservation and emulsifiers (emulsifiers are used to mix oils with water).

Because body butter is such a vague term, and companies use it to talk about a real butter, it is important to differentiate between a lotion that contains butters or a thick lotion that has nothing to do with butter except that it is thick like a butter. I have added several different examples of body butter ingredient lists to help illustrate this difference.

Here is an ingredient list for a body butter that illustrates things to avoid:

- water
- shea (*Butyrospermum parkii*) butter
- cyclopentasiloxane
- glycerin
- glyceryl stearate
- PEG-100 stearate
- cetearyl alcohol
- grape seed (*Vitis vinifera*) oil
- lanolin alcohol
- horseradish (*Moringa pterygosperma*) seed oil
- sesame (*Sesamum indicum*) oil
- honey
- Brazil nut (*Bertholletia excelsa*) oil
- cocoa (*Theobroma cacao*) butter
- fragrance

- myristamidopropyl PG-dimonium chloride phosphate
- xanthan gum
- phenethyl alcohol
- linalool
- caprylyl glycol
- hexyl cinnamal
- butylphenyl methylpropional
- tocopherol (vitamin E)
- disodium EDTA
- benzyl salicylate
- geraniol
- hydroxycitronellal
- sodium hydroxide
- isoeugenol
- caramel
- FD&C Yellow 5

Here is an ingredient list for another body butter that also illustrates things to avoid:

- water
- shea (*Butyrospermum parkii*) butter
- cocoa (*Theobroma cacao*) butter
- cyclomethicone
- glycerin
- glyceryl stearate
- PEG-100 stearate
- cetearyl alcohol
- babassu (*Orbignya oleifera*) oil
- beeswax (*Cera alba*)
- lanolin alcohol
- phenoxyethanol
- fragrance
- methylparaben
- propylparaben
- xanthan gum
- benzyl alcohol
- disodium EDTA
- sodium hydroxide
- caramel
- FD&C Yellow 5

Here is yet another ingredient list for a body butter that also illustrates things to avoid:

- water
- olive (*Olea europaea*) oil
- cyclomethicone
- cocoa (*Theobroma cacao*) butter
- shea (*Butyrospermum parkii*) butter
- glycerin
- glyceryl stearate
- PEG-100 stearate
- cetearyl alcohol
- lanolin alcohol
- phenoxyethanol
- fragrance
- methylparaben
- propylparaben
- xanthan gum
- benzyl alcohol
- disodium EDTA
- sodium hydroxide
- caramel
- chromium oxide greens

Contrast this with an ingredient list for a body butter containing helpful ingredients to look for:

- organic virgin coconut (*Cocos nucifera*) oil
- wild African shea (*Butyrospermum parkii*) butter
- organic extra virgin olive (*Olea europaea*) oil
- organic cocoa (*Theobroma cacao*) butter
- organic jojoba (*Simmondsia chinensis*) seed oil
- wild castor bean (*Ricinus communis*) oil
- natural beeswax (*Cera alba*)
- organic CO2 extracts of sea buckthorn berry (*Hippophae rhamnoides*) and rose hip (*Rosa canina*)
- rose otto (*Rosa damascena*) essential oil
- patchouli essential oil
- cardamom (*Elettaria cardamomum*) essential oil
- blood orange (*Citrus sinensis Sanguinelli*) essential oil

Alternative Options for Least Amount of Added Toxins— Body Butters

GOOD

1. Zosimos Botanicals Cucumber Melon Body Butter
2. Wild Woozle Soap Company Ile Pacifique Crème de Corps
3. Plum Hill Body Butter

BETTER

1. Magnolia Skies Whipped Body Butter: Vanilla Lavender, Patchouli Vanilla

BEST

1. Magnolia Skies Whipped Body Butter: Patchouli Bliss
2. Back Porch Soap Company Organic 100% Shea Butter
3. Badger Body Butter: Fresh Citrus, Cocoa Vanilla, Antique Rose
4. Suki Butter Cream Healing Salve
5. Sumbody 100% Shea Butter
6. Sumbody Butters with Benefits
7. Pure Body by Ahthi Shea Butter
8. Shea Radiance Citrus Pure Shea Butter
9. Lodestar Essentials Macadamia Nut Body Butter
10. Lodestar Essentials Shea Body Butter
11. Super Salve Company Mochachino Body Butter
12. Sumbody 100% Pure Virgin Wet Coconut Butter

Body Oils

Generally your skin from the neck down likes richer butters in order for it to absorb the right type of moisture. Some people prefer oils, while others use a technique called layering, first applying body oil and then sealing it with a richer lotion or butter. There are plenty of oils available that contain no harmful ingredients. Just like cooking oils with no additional ingredients, these require no preservation and have the same shelf life. You can smell the oil and determine if it has gone rancid. Rancid oils should not be used either in cooking or on your skin, as they contain free radicals. Use oils sparingly to minimize transfer to and possible staining of clothing and bed linens.

When companies start adding unnecessary ingredients such as fresh lemon and soy milk to an oil, they create a need for preservation. While these ingredients are good for your skin, they don't add anything that the oil alone cannot provide. Unfortunately, most companies use synthetic and harmful ingredients for preservation. An effective body oil does not need all the extra fluff to "combat wrinkles" or make your skin "feel silky smooth." It should naturally contain a combination of oils that can achieve the same effect without added chemicals. There are a wide variety of natural oils available that provide wonderful skin-loving properties. Rose-hip oil is naturally high in vitamin C, carrot oil is high in vitamins A and D, and avocado oil contains essential fatty acids. Additionally, the natural form of oils is generally more absorbable, and your skin can actually metabolize it more effectively.

Here is the ingredient list for a body oil that illustrates things to avoid:

- caprylic/capric triglyceride
- sweet almond (*Prunus amygdalis dulcis*) oil
- babassu (*Orbignya oleifera*) oil
- coconut (*Cocos nucifera*) oil
- perfume
- linalool
- tocopherol (vitamin E)
- hexyl cinnamal
- gardenia (*Gardenia jasminoides*)
- ylang-ylang (*Cananga odorata*)
- benzyl benzoate
- benzyl salicylate
- black pepper (*Piper nigrum*)
- geraniol
- farnesol
- jasmine (*Jasminum officinale*)
- benzyl alcohol
- limonene

- eugenol
- amyl cinnamal
- citronellal
- coumarin
- hydroxycitronellal
- isoeugenol

Contrast this with an ingredient list for a body oil containing helpful ingredients to look for:

- almond (*Prunus amygdalus*) oil
- avocado (*Persea gratissima*) oil
- olive (*Olea europaea*) oil
- essential oils of lavender (*Lavandula angustifolia*) and orange (*Citrus aurantium dulcis*)

Alternative Options for Least Amount of Added Toxins— Body Oils

GOOD

1. LaLicious Body Oil: Vanilla, Lily Mango

BETTER

1. Organic Apoteke Turkish Rose Body Hydrate Oil
2. Hugo Natural Botanical Apothecary Massage & Body Oil: Eucalyptus, French Lavender, Unscented

BEST

1. Nature's Gate Vitamin E Oil Roll-on Body Oil
2. Weleda Baby Calendula Oil
3. Weleda Pregnancy Body Oil
4. GratefulBody Midnight Oil
5. Pangea Organics Massage & Body Oil
6. Wild Woozle Soap Company Absolute Passion Massage and Body Oil
7. Wild Woozle Soap Company After Yoga Massage Oil
8. Badger Healing Birch Massage & Body Oil
9. Suki Delicate Hydrating Oil

10. Sumbody Body Oil: Avocado, Pistachio, Golden Jojoba

11. Sumbody Massage Oil: Deep Healing, Potion #9, Stress Relief

TIPS

Your skin loses the most moisture in the first five minutes after a shower or bath. Moisturize in the shower or bath, or apply moisture immediately after drying.

Drink lots of water.

Use a humidifier to add moisture to the air.

Take essential fatty acid supplements.

Add colloidal oats to your bath (read the label to be sure the product contains no drying ingredients).

Add oils to your bath (be very careful! They make the surface extremely slippery).

For severely dry hands and feet, apply a rich butter, such as shea, and wear 100 percent cotton gloves and booties when you sleep. You can also apply the butter to other dry areas and wrap with cotton cloth.

Avoid using detergent or soap unless the soap is handmade and not milled.

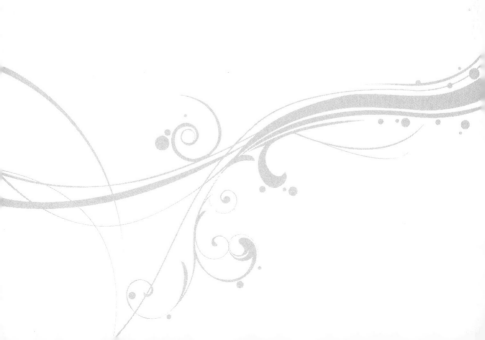

Chapter 9

The Daily Minimum

Toothpaste,
Deodorant/Antiperspirant,
and Soap

18 Consider this statement from a *U.S. News & World Report* article published in 1998: "We look good, we smell good, and we have just exposed ourselves to 200 different chemicals a day through personal-care products." Ten years later not much has changed, except perhaps the number. If it was two hundred then, how many is it now?

The products we use every day deserve a lot of attention, since these are obviously the ones we're exposed to the most frequently. These are the products we use primarily to keep our bodies clean, keep ourselves feeling fresh, and prevent health problems. We each have our own individual daily minimum; these are just the bare basics. If there are other products that you use every day, such as shampoo, face cream, or body lotion, you should pay close attention to those as well.

Toothpaste

For years I used what I believed to be an all-natural toothpaste, until I realized it was no different from the brands I was trying to avoid. I told myself it was at least better because it was made by a small family-run business. Even that was wrong; the company had been sold to one of the very companies that manufactures the other brands. Following this realization, I made one of those "I can't be perfect" decisions: I let go of my toothpaste dilemma and just used whatever my daughters brought home.

This was working well for me (a little denial goes a long way), since I thought I had no options, until my daughter asked me to pick up toothpaste for her. She wanted mint-flavored baking soda toothpaste. That sounded simple enough, until I was standing in front of the toothpaste display in my local drugstore. There was baking soda mint paste, baking soda mint gel, baking soda with peroxide gel, baking soda with peroxide non-gel, mint, super mint, wintermint, cool mint, and the list went on. The number of choices was mind-numbing. In my confusion I called my daughter, who was equally confused, and then just grabbed a box. Standing there, I realized just how far these companies go to get our dollars.

I don't know much about manufacturing toothpaste, but after ten minutes in the toothpaste aisle, I could see that it is very similar to manufacturing the products I manufacture. I'm convinced there is little difference between toothpastes except the "active" ingredients and the taste. They have one of two bases, gel or paste, and the rest is all marketing. It is the three-second buzz—the white-teeth, anti-plaque promise—that grabs you, and the five-second reading of the box that seals the deal. With so many choices and so much jargon, it is important to have a basic knowledge of some of the ingredients—especially the ones you want to avoid.

Added to strengthen our enamel, fluoride is recommended by dentists and is a component of most toothpastes on the market. A study prepared by U.K. Medicines Information (UKMi) pharmacists for National Health Service professionals delves into the potential harms of fluoride in toothpaste. Fluoride has not been proven to pose a significant threat if used three times daily in toothpaste and spit out completely. If this were the end of the story, everything would be dandy. However, toothpaste is not the only product that contains fluoride, which means we must consider the effect of the total amount we are being exposed to when evaluating the potential harms. Most tap water contains small amounts of fluoride, as do some infant formulas. These are the three main sources of fluoride in the United States. The infant formulas are especially scary because while the standard for a toxic level of consumption for an adult male in the United States is ten milligrams per day, there is no standard for young children. Given this information, I would suggest that parents try to limit their children's fluoride consumption. While flavored toothpastes such as strawberry, banana, and bubble gum encourage children to brush their teeth, they also encourage them to eat their toothpaste. Excessive ingestion of fluoride can lead to enamel fluorosis, swelling, redness, irritation, and many other adverse and potentially fatal effects. Studies suggest that children under the age of seven should not use toothpaste with fluoride.

Toothpaste often also contains sodium lauryl sulfate, dyes, and many other chemicals.

Here is an ingredient list for a toothpaste that illustrates things to avoid:

Active ingredient:

- stannous fluoride 0.454% (0.16% fluoride ion)

Inactive ingredients:

- glycerin
- hydrated silica
- sodium hexametaphosphate
- propylene glycol
- PEG-6
- water
- zinc lactate
- trisodium phosphate
- artificial flavor
- sodium lauryl sulfate
- sodium gluconate
- carrageenan
- sodium saccharin
- polyethylene
- xanthan gum
- titanium dioxide
- FD&C Blue 1

Contrast this with an ingredient list for a toothpaste containing helpful ingredients to look for:

- filtered water
- calcium carbonate
- guar gum
- certified organic mint oil
- certified organic tea tree (*Melaleuca alternifolia*) oil
- no sodium lauryl sulfate and fluoride. With organic ingredients, made in the United States, all natural, vegetarian, handmade, chemical-free, cruelty-free, never tested on animals

Alternative Options for Least Amount of Added Toxins— Toothpaste

| GOOD

1. Jasön Healthy Mouth Tea Tree Toothpaste: Tea Tree & Cinnamon
2. Auromère Herbal Toothpaste (contains sodium lauryl sulfate, but it is lower on the ingredient list than in other toothpastes)

| BETTER

1. Burt's Bees Toothpaste

| BEST

1. Miessence Toothpaste: Lemon, Mint

> **TIP** Choose mint toothpaste to help keep your breath fresh and combat bacteria.

Deodorant and Antiperspirant

Deodorant and antiperspirant have gotten a lot of press lately because there's been some concern over whether they are linked to breast cancer in women. While experts still disagree, this debate has caused a budding awareness in consumers. However, breast cancer is not the only concern when it comes to antiperspirant. To prevent sweating, it clogs pores, which causes more moisture and creates a vicious cycle. You have to use more antiperspirant in order to combat the increase in sweat production and odor. I call this the cosmetic conundrum. There is no natural antiperspirant that will work as well as the chemical product, and you shouldn't need one—bodies need to sweat. However, there are many great deodorants on the market that effectively combat odor and can also reduce perspiration to some degree.

Most people start using deodorant or antiperspirant in their teenage or preteen years when their hormones kick in and create body odor and excess sweat. If you talk with your child and find an alternative that they feel comfortable with, it will reduce sweat and odor in the long run. Once people pass through their teenage years, if they have not used antiperspirants or gobs of chemicals in their deodorant, the odor dissipates naturally. Natural alternatives include sprays, roll-ons, bars, and essential oils that help kill the bacteria that cause body odor. These come in a variety of scents and packages, and with a bit of effort you should be able to find one that is effective and that your child is comfortable using. For adults, the switch may take a little longer. You will go through a detoxification period during which you will produce more body odor and sweat more profusely because your body is purging the chemicals. Give yourself a few months to live with it and work through it, and when you come out on the other end, your body will be cleaner, purified, and smell and sweat less. There are other factors that affect body odor, such as diet and exercise, so if you have severe body odor, you should look into changing your habits. You need to deal with it, not mask it, in order to prevent body odor from worsening in the long run.

When it comes to finding a good natural product, focus on a blend of antibacterial essential oils that does not contain fragrance. One note: As I was researching deodorants and antiperspirants, I was shocked to find the word *fragrance* in Weleda's deodorant. Further research taught me that this refers only to essential oils. The reason it is called a fragrance on the label is because labeling laws are different in Europe and even Weleda's products for the United States adhere to those standards. Additionally, ingredients such as linalool, limonene, and other naturally occurring components are not separate ingredients, but rather naturally occurring molecules within essential oils. Again, this is something that only has to be declared for sale in the European Union. I mention this because in the United States linalool and limonene have ratings of nine on the Skin Deep website and essential oils have ratings of one to three. I don't want someone to look at Skin Deep and choose not to use Weleda products, many of which I consider safe.

Aside from those tidbits, one of the most widely acclaimed and trusted natural deodorants (if you can't handle the smell of strong essential oils) is the crystal rock, which, despite its name, comes in bar, roll-on, crystal rock, and spray forms.

While deodorant and antiperspirant might seem like something that you'd just rather stick with using the chemicals for, chemicals are actually more dangerous in these products than in many other products. This is especially true for women because deodorant and antiperspirant are applied so close to breast tissue, and many of the most common deodorant ingredients have been found in breast-cancer tissue.

Here is an ingredient list for a deodorant that illustrates things to avoid:

Active ingredient:
- aluminum zirconium tetrachlorohydrex glycene (18.5%)

Inactive ingredients:
- cyclopentasiloxane
- stearyl alcohol
- PPG-14 butyl ether
- dimethicone
- C12-15 alkyl benzoate
- hydrogenated castor (*Ricinus communis*) bean oil
- talc
- fragrance (perfume)
- sunflower oil (*Helianthus annuus*)
- steareth-100
- vegetable oil (olus)
- glyceryl oleate
- glycerin
- propylene glycol
- butylated hydroxytoluene (BHT)
- t-butyl hydroquinone
- citric acid

Contrast this with an ingredient list for a deodorant containing helpful ingredients to look for:
- distilled water
- witch hazel (*Hamamelis virginiana*) extract distillate
- aloe vera (*Aloe barbadensis*) juice
- organic grape alcohol
- mineral salts
- pure essential oil blend

Alternative Options for Least Amount of Added Toxins— Deodorant

| GOOD

1. Dr. Hauschka Deodorant

| BETTER

1. Lafe's Natural Hemp Oil Roll-On Deodorant
2. Home Health Herbal Magic Roll-On Deodorant

BEST

1. Miessence Aroma-Free Roll-On Deodorant
2. Botanical Skin Works Herbal Body Deodorant
3. Burt's Bees Herbal Deodorant
4. Benedetta Deodorant
5. Sumbody Be Fresh Body Deodorant

TIP Watch your diet to minimize your body's odor. Aim for lots of vegetables, especially ones that contain zinc (such as parsley, spinach, and collard greens), and drink plenty of water, while reducing consumption of garlic, red meat, and coffee.

Soap

There are two main types of soap, liquid gel and bar. For information on liquid gel soap, refer to Chapter 11 on body/hand wash. Bar soap comes in three basic types: glycerin soaps, detergent and milled soaps, and old-fashioned handmade soaps. Glycerin soaps are clear and often colorful, with designs and colored chunks. During World War II, soap manufacturers realized that if they extracted all the glycerin from the soap they were manufacturing, they could increase their profits by selling the glycerin to the weapons industry (for use as an ingredient in explosives) for a much higher price than they would get for it if they sold it in soap. This extraction left only the detergent, which the companies sold to the public as soap. True glycerin is good for your skin, but it is milky, as opposed to translucent. Modern companies use chemicals to make glycerin soap clear. Technologically, we have progressed beyond the need to create handmade soap in order to extract glycerin. Instead, companies manufacture synthetic glycerin on its own. This substance provides no benefit for your skin.

The second type of bar soap is your standard Dove or Ivory, which is made from leftover detergents. This is the same as milled soap. When manufacturers mill soap, they are removing the glycerin and leaving the detergent behind. Detergent removes your body's natural moisture, causing you to need more soap and moisturizing lotion. So don't be fooled by expensive bars that say "Triple Milled" or "French Milled"; they are still detergent.

Only pure handmade soap is truly good for your skin. This soap contains ingredients that are bonded to create a new substance (neither glycerin nor detergent), which moisturizes and cleans your skin. Natural soaps are not always as hard as synthetic soaps, and since hard soap can last longer, hardness is something consumers often look for. However, as long as natural soap is kept away from a direct spray of water, there should be very little difference in how long your bar will last compared to a synthetic, and you might be surprised how quickly you become accustomed to the softer bar.

While handmade soap is more expensive, it decreases your need for moisturizers and helps end the cosmetic conundrum caused by synthetic soaps. It also feels better on your skin. With soap, it is easy to see the difference between chemical and natural. Take a bath or shower and wash one half of your body with regular drugstore detergent soap and the other half with natural handmade soap. When you get out of the shower, feel each arm. The one you washed with detergent will feel dry and may squeak when you run a finger over it, hence the term "squeaky clean." The arm you washed with the natural soap will feel soft, supple, and moisturized. Good soaps abound, and they feel and smell as good as, or better than, chemical ones. Using a natural soap is one of the simplest ways to decrease your exposure to chemicals.

Here is an ingredient list for a soap that illustrates things to avoid:

- organic sodium palmate
- sodium palmate
- water
- organic sodium cocoate
- glycerin
- sodium
- palm kernelate
- perfume
- shea (*Butyrospermum parkii*) butter
- organic honey
- pentasodium pentetate
- tetrasodium etidronate

- sodium chloride
- tetrasodium EDTA

Contrast this with an ingredient list for a soap containing helpful ingredients to look for:

- saponified oils of olive (*Olea europaea*), coconut (*Cocos nucifera*), palm (*Elaeis guineensis*), and safflower (*Carthamus tinctorius*)
- essential oils of lavender (*Lavandula angustifolia*) and peppermint (*Mentha piperita*)

Alternative Options for Least Amount of Added Toxins— Soap

There are so many options for the "Best" category here, there's no need to bother with "Good" and "Better." Soap is either "Best" or not so good—there is little in between. The only thing a good bar of handmade soap will have that would keep it off the "Best" list would be fragrance. In addition to the companies that I have listed here you should be able to find excellent soaps close to home. Look for bar soaps made only with oils that you recognize, such as olive, avocado, palm, and safflower, and pure essential oils for scent.

BEST

1. Dr. Bronner's Magic Soaps Pure Castile Bar Soap
2. Zosimos Botanicals Natural Soap
3. Badger Beauty Bar
4. Pangea Organics Bar Soap
5. Monavé Bar Soap
6. Sumbody Bar Soap
7. Sumbody Liquid Hand Wash
8. Sumbody Supernatural Body Wash
9. Plantlife Bar Soap
10. Juniper Ridge Soap
11. Sappo Hill Oatmeal Fragrance-Free Soap
12. Any brand of liquid soap that is 100 percent liquid Castile with pure essential oils

13. Magnolia Skies soaps

14. Shea Radiance soaps

15. Delights of the Earth Handmade Soap (this company is always coming out with new scents, so check the labels carefully since some have fragrance)

16. Cranberry Lane Soap Bar (look at the different scents carefully; some contain fragrance)

17. Natural Family Botanicals Handcrafted Soaps

TIPS

Lather and then rinse soap off quickly to avoid prolonged contact with skin. Focus on necessary areas such as underarms and folds of skin.

Keep pure soap out of standing water. Unlike detergent bars, pure soap can be softer and will "melt" faster in water.

Use a good lathering soap to shave with and eliminate shaving cream.

Chapter 10

Foundation, Eyes, Cheeks, and Lips

A beautiful woman should
break her mirror early.

— BALTASAR GRACIÁN Y MORALES

Presents, balloons, cake, and little girls in red lipstick with pink smeared across their cheeks—this is a typical scene at a five-year-old's birthday party. I remember coming home from work one day to find that my youngest daughter had gotten into my makeup. She had a vibrant outline of red lipstick around her mouth and ended up with about an eighth of a stick in her stomach. At that age, she was trying to emulate me, her mother. A few years later, she started to associate makeup with beauty, and she began rummaging through my makeup again, this time for different reasons. This illustrates the overwhelming prevalence of makeup in our society. From eight to eighty, many women are uncomfortable leaving the house "without their face on." This expression illustrates the extent to which we are literally uncomfortable in our own skin. The scope and popularity of cosmetics make it an important facet of the beauty industry, and many women use several products every day. A woman might use foundation, bronzer, blush, eye shadow, eyeliner, mascara, shimmer powder, lip liner, lipstick, lip gloss, and often more than one of each.

Unlike a face wash or body scrub, which we rinse off, makeup is meant to last all day. The length of contact with these products enhances their ability to leach harmful chemicals into our skin. Where we apply makeup also creates a net of exposure that is unmatched by any other type of beauty product, since these products are being applied to some of the most sensitive areas on our bodies. Our eyelids, where we apply liner and shadow, are among the thinnest membranes protecting us from the outside world. We are even less protected from the toxins in mascara, since throughout the day, tiny mascara particulates fall from our lashes into our eyes. Lipstick is arguably the worst because it goes directly onto (and into) our mouths. Studies on the lead content in lipsticks suggest that women ingest several pounds of lipstick per year. Luckily, the market for natural alternatives is burgeoning, and consumers are gaining autonomy and choice concerning their makeup purchases.

Foundation

A good foundation creates a clean canvas for makeup. For most people, it is a way to cover blemishes, unwanted freckles, or splotchy skin and create an even tone. The most important aspect of foundation is that it matches your skin, looks smooth, and does not create a ring of orange around your neck. It should not peel or appear chunky or flaky. Conventional foundations are made up of a smorgasbord of chemicals, with a bit of pigment thrown in. The pigment can be natural or unnatural. The chemicals can clog pores; cause wrinkles, dryness, and redness; and accelerate the effects of aging. Ironically, these are the symptoms most people are seeking to combat. I found a label that shocked me on a product meant to be handled by humans and used on your skin. It was on a Bobbi Brown foundation bottle. It read: "For external use only. Keep out of eyes. Rinse with water to remove. Stop use and ask a doctor if rash or irritation develops and lasts. Keep out of reach of children. If swallowed, contact a Poison Control Center or get medical help right away." Clearly, manufacturers are aware of the potential harms of their products. How can we feel comfortable using a product on our face that, if ingested, requires a visit to the Poison Control Center?

Until recently, there were very few alternatives, but the public has begun to demand natural products, and a flurry of companies has risen to the occasion. Switching to a natural brand will automatically reduce redness, dryness, wrinkles, and aging. These products can also be more effective than their chemical counterparts in terms of creating a flawless surface upon which to apply makeup. Mineral makeup is the most common type of natural cosmetic. The bonus of mineral makeup is that it eliminates the line around your neck. But don't be fooled—just because a foundation is made of minerals does not mean it is truly natural or safe. The most popular and widely recognized mineral brand uses ingredients such as bismuth oxide (natural, but not good for skin), mineral oil (petroleum), talc (carcinogenic, can be contaminated with asbestos), and fragrances.

Here is an ingredient list for a foundation that illustrates things to avoid:

- water
- cyclopentasiloxane
- isohexadecane
- cetyl PEG/PPG-10/1 dimethicone
- ethylhexyl palmitate
- pentylene glycol
- trimethylsiloxysilicate
- butylene glycol
- disteardimonium hectorite
- glyceryl ethylhexanoate/stearate/adipate
- ethylhexyl glycerin
- methicone
- disodium EDTA
- PPG-15 stearyl ether
- dipropylene glycol
- retinol palmitate
- castor (*Ricinus communis*) bean oil
- corn (*Zea mays*) oil
- xylitol
- lemon (*Citrus medica limonum*) extract
- olive (*Olea europaea*) leaf extract
- papaya (*Carica papaya*) extract
- cork oak (*Quercus suber*) bark extract

May contain:
- titanium dioxide
- iron oxides

Contrast this with an ingredient list for a foundation containing helpful ingredients to look for:

- mica
- boron nitride
- titanium dioxide
- silica microspheres
- magnesium stearate
- pearl powder
- silk powder
- shea (*Butyrospermum parkii*) butter

Alternative Options for Least Amount of Added Toxins— Foundation

Note: When it comes to makeup, I decided not to include any products under the "Good" category because most makeup that does not contain a lot of harmful ingredients still contains either bismuth oxide, a cheap natural filler that is not good for skin, or talc, and I couldn't bring myself to list any makeup with either of these ingredients. However, there are plenty of "Best" options.

BETTER

1. Musq Mineral Liquid Foundation

BEST

1. Musq Mineral Powder Foundation

2. Monavé Loose Mineral Foundation

3. Monavé Cream Foundation

4. Sumbody Mineral Foundation

5. Affordable Mineral Makeup Foundation

6. Ocean Mist Cosmetics Mineral Foundation

7. CMH Essentials Mineral Foundation

8. J.Lynne Smooth Mineral Foundation

9. Everyday Minerals Base

> **TIP** Use mineral makeup and apply in layers. Apply to your neck as well as your face, and make sure to use a good moisturizer first to ensure a smooth, natural look.

Eyes

Eye makeup includes eye shadow, liners, and mascara. Shadows are used for highlights, color, and accents. Some people will use five or more colors at once. The tissue around eyes is some of the most sensitive and fragile on the body, and powders and mascara particulates tend to fall into open eyes. Mascara poses an additional threat because it is a perfect home to bacteria that stew inside the tube. This threat is amplified by sharing mascara. Expert recommendations for when to replace mascara to decrease the risk caused by bacteria range from four to eight months. Not only are these products formulated to last all day, many people do not remove them completely before going to sleep. Mascara flakes off and eye shadows slide into eyes, creating a greater direct exposure to chemicals, accelerated signs of aging, and redness and puffiness in the morning.

Health concerns about makeup pop up daily. A May 22, 2008, article in *The New York Times* warned of the hazards of mascara. Whether natural or synthetic, all makeup should be completely removed at the end of the day. The most natural type of eye makeup usually comes in powdered form, because creams and pressed powders require more chemicals to hold them together and create an appealing consistency.

Mascara

Here is an ingredient list for a mascara that illustrates things to avoid:

- water
- paraffin
- stearic acid
- PPG-17/IPDI/DMPA copolymer
- carnauba (*Copernicia cerifera*) wax
- beeswax (*Cera alba*)
- cyclopentasiloxane
- glyceryl stearate
- triethanolamine
- tricontanyl PVP
- gum arabic (*Acacia senegal*)
- nylon-12
- panthenol
- aloe (*Aloe barbadensis*) leaf juice
- tocopherol (vitamin E) acetate
- magnesium ascorbyl phosphate
- retinol palmitate
- dimethiconol
- lecithin
- polyethylene
- polytetrafluoroethylene (PTFE)
- diglycol/CHDM/isophthalates/SIP copolymer
- simethicone

- hydroxyethyl cellulose
- propylene glycol stearate
- propylene methylparaben
- propylparaben
- diazolidinyl urea

May contain:
- iron oxides
- titanium dioxide

Contrast this with an ingredient list for a mascara containing helpful ingredients to look for:

- water
- alcohol
- jojoba (*Simmondsia chinensis*) seed oil
- castor (*Ricinus communis*) bean oil
- carnauba (*Copernicia cerifera*) wax
- cetyl alcohol
- emulsifying wax NF
- glycerin
- gum arabic (*Acacia senegal*)
- stearic acid
- mica
- iron oxides
- pomelo (*Citrus grandis*) seed extract

Eye Shadow

Here is an ingredient list for an eye shadow that illustrates things to avoid:

- boron nitride
- dimethicone
- talc
- cyclopentasiloxane
- polypropylene
- trimethylsiloxysilicate
- nylon-12
- acrylates/dimethicone copolymer
- zinc stearate
- cetyl alcohol
- dimethicone

- butylene glycol dicaprylate
- acrylates copolymer
- silica
- methicone
- mineral oil
- phenoxyethanol
- methylparaben
- ethylparaben
- propylparaben

May contain:

- mica
- bismuth oxychloride
- iron oxides
- titanium dioxide
- ultramarine
- carmine
- manganese violet
- chromium hydroxide green
- ferric ferrocyanide
- FD&C Blue 1
- FD&C Yellow 5
- FD&C Red 40

Contrast this with an ingredient list for an eye shadow containing helpful ingredients to look for:

- mica
- iron oxides
- titanium dioxide

Alternative Options for Least Amount of Added Toxins— Mascara and Eye Shadow

GOOD

1. Miessence Mascara

2. Monavé Mascara

3. Real Purity Mascara

BETTER

1. Beauty Wise Mineral Mascara

BEST

1. Jasco Organics makeup, all products (at time of review)
2. Musq Musqhave Mineral Mascara
3. Musq Eyeliner Kohl Pencil
4. Zosimos Botanicals eyeshadows eye pencils
5. Musq Eye Shadow, all colors (at time of review)
6. Affordable Mineral Makeup Eye Shadow or Liner, all products (at time of review)
7. Monavé Ultra-Mattes for Eyes
8. Sumbody Mineral Eye Shadow
9. Affordable Mineral Makeup Eyeliner Pencil
10. CMH Essentials Eye Shadow
11. J.Lynne Eye Shadow
12. Everyday Minerals Eye Shadow

TIPS

Curl lashes and use less mascara. Apply mascara to only your top lashes and replace product every two to three months to avoid bacteria growth.

Wet makeup brush and use mineral makeup on your eyes for a more dramatic look.

Multitask with your colors. Use soft pinks, browns, peaches, and mauve on both lids and cheeks.

Use mineral makeup and replace eye pencils with a precision brush and a dark eye shadow. This eliminates the creases caused by eye pencils and cuts down on the amount of makeup you purchase.

Cheeks

The good news about blush is that it is applied to a relatively small area, and it doesn't fall into your eyes or creep into your mouth. The bad news is it still seeps through your skin—but the exposure is much less than that of eye or lip makeup. If you develop any sort of rash or breakout where you apply blush, you'll know what's causing it. Some people wear a darker blush, or bronzer, all over the face, in which case the same hazards from exposure to foundation apply. There are several good options for natural blush on the market.

Here is an ingredient list for a blush that illustrates things to avoid:

- ethylhexyl palmitate
- hydrogenated polyisobutene
- nylon-12
- isodecyl neopentanoate
- microcrystalline wax (*cera microcristallina*)
- isopropyl lanolin
- carnauba (*Copernicia cerifera*) wax
- talc
- acrylates copolymer
- shea (*Butyrospermum parkii*) butter
- dimethicone
- methylparaben

May contain:

- iron oxides
- mica
- titanium dioxide
- D&C Red 7

Contrast this with an ingredient list for a blush containing helpful ingredients to look for:

- mica
- iron oxides
- titanium dioxide

Alternative Options for Least Amount of Added Toxins— Cheeks

| BEST

1. Jasco Organics Fresh Look Blush
2. Affordable Mineral Makeup Blush
3. Musq Musqskin Gilding Bronzer
4. Musq Musqskin Gilding Blush

5. Monavé Blush

6. Monavé Bronzer

7. Sumbody Blush

8. Sumbody Bronzer

9. CMH Essentials Blush/Bronzer

10. J.Lynne Soft Silk Mineral Blush

11. Earth's Beauty Blush (some colors contain carmine)

12. Everyday Minerals Blush

> **TIP** Use mineral makeup and choose three blush colors. Use your highlight color for an eyelid cover, your basic color for an eye shadow, and a contour color that can double as a bronzer. With mineral makeup you can also mix and match, so don't be afraid to try new things!

Lips

Lipsticks, liners, and glosses have the most direct route into your body—via your mouth. The debate is still raging over the number of pounds of lipstick the average woman ingests per year. On October 11, 2007, the Campaign for Safe Cosmetics issued a press release reporting that an independent lab tested thirty-three brands of lipstick sold in the United States and 60 percent contained potentially hazardous levels of lead. In an effort to change the color of our lips, we are unknowingly and without consent eating lead. While lead is probably the most harmful substance found in lipsticks, many lipsticks also contain tallow (animal fat), E120 (crushed insects) for coloring, and a plethora of chemicals. So when you're all dressed up and out at a fancy restaurant and you detect an aphid on your salad, relax and enjoy your meal, knowing that the aphid is in good company.

Here is an ingredient list for a lipstick that illustrates things to avoid:

Active ingredients:

• allantoin (0.6%)

• octinoxate (7.5%)

Inactive ingredients:

- diisopropyl dimer dilinoleate
- hydrogenated polyisobutene
- polyglyceryl-2 diisostearate
- octyldodecanol
- BIS-diglyceryl polyacyladipate-2
- polyethylene
- squalene
- jojoba (*Simmondsia chinensis*) seed oil
- ozokerite
- microcrystalline wax (*Cera microcristallina*)
- shea (*Butyrospermum parkii*) butter
- VP/hexadecane copolymer
- silica
- tocopherol (vitamin E) acetate
- PEG-5 rapeseed sterol
- alumina
- disteardimonium hectorite
- fragrance
- isopropyl paraben
- butylparaben
- isobutylparaben
- glyceryl stearate SE
- behenyl alcohol
- pentaerythrityl tetraisostearate
- palmitic acid
- stearic acid
- butylated hydroxytoluene (BHT)
- propylene carbonate
- synthetic fluorphogopite
- C12-16 alcohols
- calcium aluminum borosilicate
- calcium sodium borosilicate
- ascorbyl palmitate (vitamin C)
- lecithin
- tin oxide
- silica
- dimethyl silylate
- polyethylene terephthalate
- polymethyl methacrylate

- aluminum hydroxide
- sodium chondroitin sulfate
- atelocollagen
- dimethicone

May contain:

- mica
- titanium dioxide
- iron oxides
- D&C Red 7
- FD&C Yellow 6
- D&C Red 28
- FD&C Yellow 5
- FD&C Blue 1
- carmine
- D&C Red 36

Contrast this with an ingredient list for a lipstick containing helpful ingredients to look for:

- castor (*Ricinus communis*) bean oil
- jojoba (*Simmondsia chinensis*) seed oil
- mica
- carnauba (*Copernicia cerifera*) wax
- candelilla (*Euphorbia antisyphilitica*) wax
- shea (*Butyrospermum parkii*) butter
- orange (*Citrus aurantium dulcis*) peel oil
- tocopherol (vitamin E)
- iron oxides
- titanium dioxide

Lip Balm

Many people call this ChapStick, which is a brand name. The generic term for the typically colorless salve for moisturizing lips is lip balm. Lips are exposed to sun, wind, and cold without the shield of clothing. It is no wonder they often become dry and chapped. Unlike most other lip products, lip balm is used by everyone from small children to grown adults. As with other lip products, we inadvertently consume small amounts of lip balm, so it is important to find a natural version.

Some all-natural lip balms are more effective than others. Cocoa butter is a commonly used ingredient, and while it is perfectly safe, it is not the best moisturizing agent for lips. Instead, look for products containing large quantities of shea butter, which deeply moisturizes lips. Lip balm is no exception to the chemical conundrum—many people feel they are addicted to their lip balm. This is because some lip balms, especially those stewed with chemicals, feel great as long as you're using them but dry out your skin as soon as you neglect or stop using them, making you even more reliant on them. The main reason for this is a mixture of chemicals and a high concentration of synthetic wax. Usually the harder the balm, the more wax. This wax acts like a protective coating to make your lips feel moisturized when it is on but leaves them chapped and red when it wears off. Mixed with chemicals that dry your skin and lacking a proper hydrating agent, these balms only harm your lips further. A good lip balm should enrich the moisture content of your lips without creating an addiction. Some of the most important harmful ingredients to avoid when purchasing a lip balm are petroleum-based products and preservatives. With that advice, go out and look for a lip balm that makes your lips feel as great after you use it as when you put it on.

Here is an ingredient list for a lip balm that illustrates things to avoid:

Active ingredients:
- octyl dimethyl PABA (8%)
- octinoxate (7.5%)
- oxybenzone (6%)
- homosalate (5%)
- sunscreen
- dimethicone (1.1%)

Inactive ingredients:
- allantoin
- aloe (*Aloe barbadensis*) leaf extract
- beeswax (*Cera alba*)
- butylparaben
- coconut (*Cocos nucifera*) oil
- candelilla (*Euphorbia antisyphilitica*)wax

- fragrance
- isopropyl paraben
- isocetyl alcohol
- isobutylparaben
- methylparaben
- myristyl lactate
- ozokerite
- panthenol
- petrolatum
- castor (*Ricinus communis*) bean oil
- silica
- cocoa (*Theobroma cacao*) butter
- tocopherol (vitamin E)

Contrast this with an ingredient list for a lip balm containing helpful ingredients to look for:

- extra virgin olive (*Olea europaea*) oil
- golden yellow beeswax (*Cera alba*)
- castor (*Ricinus communis*) bean oil
- extract of aloe vera (*Aloe barbadensis*)
- rose hip (*Rosa canina*) seed C02 extract
- extract of sea buckthorn berry (*Hippophae rhamnoides*)

Alternative Options for Least Amount of Toxins—Lipstick and Lip Gloss

BETTER

1. Kiss My Face 3-Way Color (for Lips, Cheeks, and Eyes)

2. Honeybee Gardens Truly Natural Lipstick

BEST

1. Jasco Organics Fresh Look Vegan Lipstick

2. Miessence Lip Crème

3. Badger Classic Lip Balm: Vanilla Madagascar, Pink Grapefruit, Lavender & Orange, Tangerine Breeze, Highland Mint, Ginger & Lemon, Unscented

4. Suki Lip Repair Butter

5. Wild Woozle Soap Company Namaste Lip Care

6. Musq Moisturizing Mineral Lipstick
7. Monavé Lip Liner
8. Monavé Liquid Gloss
9. Monavé Lip Gloss
10. Monavé Lip Tip, Lip Glaze, Lipstick, Lip Crayon
11. Sumbody Eye Shadow (doubles as lip color when mixed with lip balm)
12. Sumbody Lucky Lips Lip Balm (mix with Sumbody Eye Shadow for color)
13. Natural Family Botanicals Herbal Lip Heal
14. Delights of the Earth Liberated Lips Lip Balm
15. Natural Family Botanicals Shea Butter Lip Tint
16. J.Lynne Lip Smooth Color Lip Cream
17. Primitive Lipstick
18. Eco Lip Eco Tint
19. Everyday Minerals Lip Gloss

TIPS

Mix a mineral blush with lip balm for an innovative lipstick. Always apply lip balm first to moisturize and smooth lips.

Use natural lip balms around your cuticles to prevent tearing and abrasions as well as to strengthen and condition nails and help them grow.

Chapter 11

Shampoo and Conditioner, Body Wash, Hand Wash, and Shower Gel

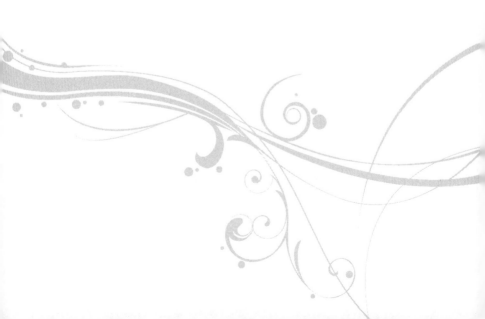

Sinking into a deep tub of soft bubbles that dance into the air, reflecting gold from the bathtub fixtures—this is one of the most iconic scenes of luxury in our culture. We are obsessed with lather, bubbles, and foam. Tallow has been used for centuries to produce a natural lather for a bar soap, but not only is it not the best thing for your skin, many consumers are turned off by the idea of bathing in animal products. This leaves manufacturers with very little choice but to employ a synthetic alternative. The most common surfactant—an ingredient that causes lather—until recently was sodium lauryl sulfate. When it began receiving pervasive bad press and consumers became savvy about its harms, manufacturers had to switch. It is now commonplace to see products that advertise "no sodium lauryl sulfate." While this appears to be good news, it can in fact be the opposite, because consumers are unaware that many chemicals used to replace sodium lauryl sulfate, such as cocamidopropyl betaine, pose all of the same, if not more, threats. Because consumers are so accustomed to chemical lathers, it is extremely difficult to create a lather without chemicals that can match those standards. Many companies that call their products "natural" claim soap root or yucca as their source of lather, but I have tried these in my lab, and without another (chemical) lathering agent, they don't produce the type of lather we desire.

On a positive note, each generation of new natural ingredients gets better (more natural). As the public demands safer options, more raw ingredients to produce cleaner products become available. As of this writing, I am currently using the best surfactant I can find in my shampoo and body wash. I do this at a price. Other manufacturers do not choose to use the purest ingredients they can find because it is just too cost-prohibitive. A surfactant that is more natural will cost a manufacturer between four and eight dollars per pound, compared with as little as pennies per pound for more commonly used surfactants. The surfactant I am using is forty dollars per pound. Using such expensive raw ingredients cuts into profit margins considerably. As long as the consumer is happy and is buying what a manufacturer is producing, the typical manufacturer will see no need to spend the extra money and make the change.

An important thing to remember when using these products is that it is not the lather that cleans. You can get clean hair and skin without the lather we all adore.

In some of the following categories, there are few natural options available. Because of the difficulty of finding truly safe and natural shampoos and conditioners, I was tempted to turn the "Good," "Better," "Best" list into the "Best I Could Find" list. I was not able to find the same level of purity available for most other products, so my standards had to change, but rest assured, the products listed are the best available options. I imagine in a few years the market will expand, as consumers and manufacturers start demanding healthful alternatives. Informed consumers force the raw-ingredient manufacturers to come up with better, cleaner, greener alternatives. Don't be fooled by a chemical cousin—demand truly natural products.

Shampoo and Conditioner

Although shampoo and conditioner are in the wash-off category, they still pose a great risk for exposure because of where they are applied. They are made to be scrubbed into our hair and onto our scalp—the barrier between the outside world and the capillaries that surround the brain. This is like inviting all of the chemicals and dyes from your shampoo right into your brain for a tea party and a little ransacking. Surfactants are not the only harmful ingredients found in shampoos. Chemicals closely regulate the consistency, pearl (a pearly luster), color, texture, smoothness, and other factors that define a good shampoo or conditioner. As we rinse the shampoo out of our hair, the chemicals cascade over our entire bodies and absorb through our skin. Then we stand or soak in the excess product, depending on whether we are taking a shower or bath, and we absorb even more toxins.

Each new generation of ingredients gets better as the public demand for truly natural products increases. However, consumers have to put a lot of pressure on companies to affect this change. For example, the surfactant I'm using in my shampoo has only been available for about a year. It is the best available, and believe me, I've done my detective work. I have a hard time believing in my surfactant: Why does it lather? I spoke with chemists at the company that created this surfactant. The only reason this product hasn't been taken off on the market is that while most "natural" surfactants cost between four and eight dollars per pound, this one costs forty dollars per pound. The manufacturer said he was having a hard time getting companies to buy it because they are unwilling to spend the extra money as long as their customers are happy thinking what they use is natural.

Here is an ingredient list for a shampoo that illustrates things to avoid:

- water
- sodium laureth sulfate
- coco-betaine
- glyceryl stearate SE
- avocado (*Persea gratissima*) oil
- nettle (*Urtica dioica*) leaf extract
- ammonium lauryl sulfate
- cocamide MEA
- guar hydroxypropyltrimonium chloride
- polyquaternium-7
- polyquaternium-11
- glycerin
- PEG-150 distearate
- tetrasodium EDTA
- citric acid
- sodium chloride
- phenoxyethanol
- methylparaben
- sodium benzoate
- FD&C Yellow 5
- FD&C Yellow 6
- limonene
- fragrance

Contrast this with an ingredient list for a shampoo containing helpful ingredients to look for:

- organic aloe vera (*Aloe barbadensis*) leaf juice
- cocopolyglucose
- yucca (*Yucca schidigera*) extract
- organic safflower (*Carthamus tinctorius*) seed oil
- organic avocado (*Persea gratissima*) oil
- non-GMO xanthan gum
- lime (*Citrus aurantifolia*) essential oil
- honeysuckle (*Lonicera* sp.) extract
- citric acid
- organic horsetail (*Equisetum arvense*) extract
- organic nettle (*Urtica dioica*) extract
- organic burdock (*Arctium lappa*) extract
- organic rosemary (*Rosmarinus officinalis*) extract
- organic sage (*Salvia officinalis*) extract

Alternative Options for Least Amount of Toxins— Shampoo/Conditioner

Shampoos

| GOOD

1. Hugo Natural Botanical Apothecary Shampoo: Lemon Verbena, Red Tea & Ylang-Ylang, French Lavender

| BETTER

1. Monavé Rosemary Lavender Shampoo
2. Kiss My Face Big Body Shampoo
3. Kiss My Face Whenever Shampoo

| BEST

1. Miessence Shampoo: Desert Flower, Lemon Myrtle
2. Botanical Skin Works Shampoo (Although I listed this as a "Best," its ingredients are confusing to me. Since I could not see anything that would make lather, I called the company to see it they left something off the label. They said the lathering agents are coconut oil and castor oil, and they stand behind that assertion, but I have tried these many times without success.)
3. Sumbody Head First Shampoo: Normal/Oily, Normal/Dry

4. Chagrin Valley Soap & Craft Company Shampoo Bar

5. Burt's Bees Rosemary Mint Shampoo Bar

6. Sumbody Bar Shampoo

Conditioners

| GOOD

1. Hugo Natural Botanical Apothecary Conditioner: Lemon Verbena, Red Tea & Ylang-Ylang, French Lavender

| BETTER

1. Kiss My Face Big Body Conditioner

2. Kiss My Face Whenever Conditioner

3. Max Green Alchemy Scalp Rescue Conditioner

| BEST

1. Monavé Conditioner

2. Miessence Shine Herbal Conditioner

3. Botanical Skin Works Leave-In Conditioner

4. Botanical Skin Works Lavender Cream Rinse

5. Sumbody Head First Conditioner: Normal/Oily, Normal/Dry

TIPS

Wet hair thoroughly before applying shampoo—this will allow you to use less.

Apply shampoo mostly to the hairline—the rest will get washed away as you rinse.

Body Wash, Hand Wash, Liquid Soap, and Shower Gel

Called by innumerable names, these three products are essentially formulated the same way for the same purpose: to cleanse skin. In terms of harmful chemicals, they have the same rap sheet as shampoo. The only good news is that there are companies, like Dr. Bronner, that have been making liquid Castile soaps for decades. Many consumers don't like Dr. Bronner's because it isn't a gel and doesn't give the same type of lather that chemical soaps give—the combination of gel and lather is nearly impossible to re-create using only natural ingredients. If you are willing to overlook this, you can use liquid Castile soap for everything from hands and bodies to dishes.

Watch out for the claim "antibacterial," especially in hand wash. This requires extra chemicals that pose a whole new slew of problems. Although an antibacterial product sounds enticing, the fact is that exposure to bacteria helps strengthen our immune systems. Antibacterial soaps can breed resistant bacteria and lower our resistance to everyday bacteria. With the surge in consumer demand for truly natural products, manufacturers and companies are looking toward more effective alternatives, and there will likely be many more on the market within the next few years.

Here is an ingredient list for a body wash that illustrates things to avoid:

- water
- petrolatum
- ammonium laureth sulfate
- ammonium lauryl sulfate
- sodium lauroamphoacetate
- lauric acid
- trihydroxystearin
- fragrance
- sodium chloride
- tocopherol (vitamin E) acetate
- guar hydroxypropyltrimonium chloride
- citric acid
- DMDM hydantoin
- sodium benzoate
- disodium EDTA
- niacinamide
- PEG-14M
- shea (*Butyrospermum parkii*) extract
- retinol palmitate
- vitamin B-3
- vitamin E
- vitamin A

Contrast this with an ingredient list for a body wash containing helpful ingredients to look for:

- Castile soap
- lavender (*Lavandula angustifolia*) essential oil

Alternative Options for Least Amount of Toxins— Body/Hand Wash and Shower Gel

GOOD

1. Hugo Natural Botanical Apothecary Shower Gel: French Lavender, Grapefruit, Geranium

BETTER

1. Intelligent Nutrients Certified Organic Total Body Cleanser

BEST

1. Pangea Organics Shower Gel

2. Pangea Organics Liquid Soap

3. Jasco Organics Pure Body Wash

4. Zosimos Botanicals Orange and Cinnamon Shower Gel

5. Lunaroma Organic Castile Shower Gel

6. Lunaroma Synergies Organic Castile Shower Gel

7. Lunaroma Foaming Organic Hand Soap

8. Sumbody Supernatural Body Wash

9. Sumbody Supernatural Hand Wash

TIP | Use Castile soap for a liquid shower gel.

Chapter 12

Babies, Kids, and Teens

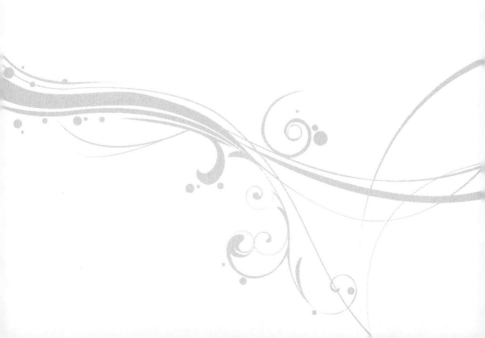

This chapter is different from the others in that it does not focus on a certain product or category of products. This is because so many products fall under this heading—and most of them are covered elsewhere in the book—that it would be impractical to create an in-depth schematic for each type. Instead, I'll discuss the overall scope of products used almost solely by babies, kids, and teens.

When we see the word *baby* on a bottle, we automatically think safe, gentle, and pure. Unfortunately, this isn't the case. When I was researching baby products, I found that the product usually contained as many harsh and toxic ingredients as the adult version. If a product is 100 percent natural—free of essential oils and questionable extracts—then chances are it is as good as or better than any product out there that happens to be labeled "baby." There are wonderful lotions made for you that would be great for your baby too, and they are probably better than those designated as baby lotions.

Every day, children are exposed to an average of twenty-seven personal-care product ingredients that have not been found safe for kids, according to a national survey conducted in 2007 by the Environmental Working Group. Overall, 77 percent of the ingredients in seventeen hundred children's products reviewed have not been assessed for safety. Besides the basics that everyone needs, babies, kids, and teens do not require many other products. However, babies and children love bath toys, bubbles, and everything fun and colorful, while teens are just being introduced to the world of adult cosmetics.

Teens are the future market for cosmetic and personal-care companies, so companies devote enormous resources to getting teens to buy their products and to ensure that they'll continue in a habit of spending money on personal-care products. Cosmetics are one of the first products teens purchase with their own money. It makes them feel grown-up and mature, and personal-care products are among the most common gifts for teens. Often, teens are attracted to bright, innovative products with cute and clever packaging. In marketing to teens, lipstick is one of the main crossover products. That means it is used to train preteens and teens to use cosmetics. My kids started out with lip balm, then moved on to sparkly glosses and finally to heavily tinted glosses and pot colors. Once a teen is using makeup, she will need makeup remover, which dries skin and creates a necessity for moisturizing creams, and all of a sudden, she is a full-fledged cosmetic consumer.

Even before beauty is on their radar, kids love to use fun bath products, and bath time creates memories that the entire family will cherish When my kids were young, I scoured the market for everything colorful, fun, new, and exciting for them to play with in the bath. Children and bath products are a natural fit, but unfortunately, most kids' products are not natural. While researching products for this book, I was astounded by the lack of entertaining natural bath products available for kids. Unfortunately, packaging labels are not enough to ensure that a product is natural. Most baby products and teen-queen kits with *natural* blasted across them are anything but. You're lucky if some of these products contain even one natural ingredient—including water.

This has inspired me to look into formulating safe alternatives. Keep an eye on the market over the next few years, and you'll find exciting new options. In an increasingly polluted environment, and with babies and kids already using soap, shampoo, and toothpaste, it is important to keep all the extras as natural and healthful as possible. And as you know now, it is especially important to be vigilant when choosing products for such delicate skin. Make good choices for your children when they're young in order to lessen their exposure over a lifetime, and teach them the practice of choosing natural products.

Bubble Bath

When talking about babies, kids, and teens it is impossible to ignore bubble bath. It is one of the most common culprits in the baby, children, and teen category. It even crosses over into the adult market in a big way. A bubble bath is the epitome of relaxation, but it means soaking in chemicals that slowly leach into our bodies. While we're talking about kids and bubble bath, forget merely the slow leaching; kids often end up eating the bubbles and drinking some of the bathwater! You have to ask yourself, "Would I feed this to my child?" When my kids were young, picking a bubble bath was one of our favorite rituals. We had Pixie Blossom and Dragon, and each one came in a beautifully illustrated seed packet. Unfortunately, after it was too late to make a difference for my kids, I learned that these bubble baths contained parabens, sodium lauryl sulfate, PEGs, and a variety of other harmful ingredients.

While my children never had a visible reaction to these chemicals, many children do. I recently read a website filled with parental concerns about bubble bath, including reports of rashes and skin irritation. Bubble bath can be especially harmful to females, who can contract vaginal infections or irritation, redness, and swelling due to prolonged contact with these chemicals. I have been trying to formulate a completely safe and natural bubble bath for at least five years, and while I can create bubbles and lather, I have not yet gotten to the point of being able to fill a bathtub with mountains of bubbles. At this point, I suggest that you forget bubble bath; fizzers and bath toys can be just as much fun, with no risk to your health or that of your child.

Here is an ingredient list for a bubble bath that illustrates things to avoid:

- water
- disodium laureth sulfosuccinate
- sodium laureth sulfate
- cocamide MEA
- aloe (*Aloe barbadensis*) leaf juice
- hydroxyethyl cellulose
- fragrance
- DMDM hydantoin
- tetrasodium EDTA
- citric acid
- D&C Red 33

Teen Body Wash

Here is an ingredient list for a teen body wash that illustrates things to avoid:

- water
- sodium laureth sulfate
- cocamidopropyl betaine
- cocamidopropyl hydroxysultaine
- sodium chloride
- glycerin
- propylene glycol
- fragrance
- polyquaternium-10
- tetrasodium EDTA
- PEG-150 distearate
- citric acid
- etidronic acid
- DMDM hydantoin
- iodopropynyl butylcarbamate
- D&C Red 33

Contrast this with an ingredient list for a teen body wash containing helpful ingredients to look for:

- Castile soap
- lavender (*Lavandula angustifolia*) essential oil

Alternative Options for Least Amount of Toxins—Baby, Kid, and Teen Products

I haven't listed any teen products below because I couldn't find any that met my criteria. I would love to be able to find some to list in the future.

This list in the baby-to-teen category is a sampling of safe products that I could find. You do not need to choose a product with a baby on the label to use it on your child. I suggest choosing from the products in the main list and ignore the marketing ploy that tells you should buy different products for your children. If it is clean, it is clean, with or without the baby on the label.

| GOOD

1. Rainbow De-Tangler for Kids

2. California Baby Non-Burning & Calming Diaper Area Wash

3. Baby Avalon Organics Protective A, D & E Ointment (contains

tribehenin, which enhances penetration, thereby increasing the ease with which chemicals can enter the bloodstream)

▌ BETTER

1. Botanical Skin Works Calendula Baby Lotion

▌ BEST

1. Earth's Best Baby Oil by Jason
2. Weleda Calendula Diaper Care
3. Weleda Baby Tummy Oil
4. Jasco Organics Baby Hugs Baby Lotion
5. Botanical Skin Works Baby Lavender Bath (although I am concerned about the apparent lack of a lathering agent)
6. Botanical Skin Works Baby Powder
7. Botanical Skin Works Baby Massage Oil
8. Botanical Skin Works Baby Bottom Ointment
9. Baby Avalon Moisturizing Organic Massage Oil
10. Badger Baby Balm
11. Badger Baby Oil
12. Lunaroma Baby's Soothing Bath
13. Lunaroma Baby's Soothing Massage Oil
14. Alba Un-Petroleum Multi-purpose Jelly
15. Botanical Skin Works Basic Natural Jelly
16. Sumbody Baby Be Moist Petroleum-Free Oil
17. Sumbody Splish Splash Baby Bath
18. Sumbody Kid Fizzer: Grumps Away!, Go to Bed Sleepyhead, Tummy Tame
19. Sumbody Bottom's Up Baby Butt Salve
20. Sumbody Baby Dew: Tiny Hiny, Dew Sleep, Dew Laugh
21. Sumbody Ooh Baby Natural Soap
22. Sumbody Little One Talc-Free Baby Powder

TIPS

Avoid bubble bath. Choose safer options for your children's bath, such as bath fizzers and bath salts.

Instead of filling the bath with bubbles—and chemicals—try this fun alternative: Make a kids' bath lab. Fill small containers with ingredients like sea salts, flower petals (think lavender, mint, rose), honey, milk, and baking soda. Put them on a tray with measuring spoons, plastic bowls, and spoons and watch your child create! This activity is not only fun, but each ingredient is safe, healthy, and good for skin.

Remember that babies, children, and teens do not need a lot of products, so keep the basics and toss the rest.

Chapter 13

Face and Eye Creams, Serums, and Oils

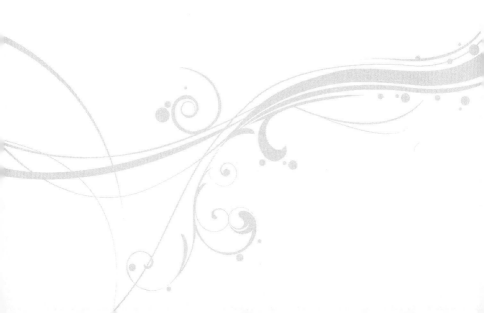

Outside of the daily necessities such as toothpaste, shampoo, and soap, face creams are the biggest sellers in the personal-care industry. Companies know that we will pay anything to look and feel younger. There is always a new "miracle" cream or revolutionary ingredient hitting the market. Because there is such a demand and so many options, it is confusing for consumers to look beyond the marketing promises and determine which product is right for them. Companies are all vying to get your dollars, making promises about everything from erasing wrinkles to restoring parched skin. The truth is, there's little difference from one brand of chemical-based face-care products to another. The most significant variable is the price of the packaging; most of the raw ingredients cost about the same. Natural face-care products differ, though, in that they can yield all the benefits we look for without any of the adverse side effects.

Face creams target unwanted skin issues and combat dry skin. There are many causes for dry skin. As we age, our skin changes. Our oil-producing glands are less active, our dead skin cells turn over more slowly, our epidermis is thinner and more fragile, and we lose the fat layer in our skin that gives it that plump, youthful appearance. Other common drying causes include sun, wind, cold weather, and most soaps, cleansers, lotions, and bath soaks. Some of the symptoms people experience with dry skin are tightness that is exaggerated after showering or swimming; a loss of plumpness; roughness; itching, flaking, or scaling; cracks or peeling; and severe redness.

These uncomfortable and sometimes unsightly side effects of dry skin make people willing to try any number of the face products available, in an attempt to find a solution. Unfortunately, in the case of both wrinkles and dry skin, most of what is in the chemical-based products does not repair or reduce these issues—it only exaggerates and exacerbates them. So we try more products. When you use natural products, your skin will show you the difference—you will no longer have to use a face cream to cover up the effects of your face cream.

Additionally, more and more people are becoming "sensitive" to face-care products. One reason for this heightened sensitivity is the ingredients used in skin-care products. Simply reducing your exposure to harmful ingredients will help maintain healthy, glowing, hydrated, youthful skin.

Face Creams

Face creams have a vast range of uses and results, the most important being the rehydration of skin. The rest of the promises made on the labels of these products range from erasing wrinkles to decreasing sagginess. If your cream can deliver on any of these claims, it is a bonus.

The difference between natural and chemical-based products in face creams is enormous. Chemical-based products might not even contain any real oils or active ingredients. They are a chemical soup, mixed to make your skin feel soft, supple, and hydrated. The only ingredients making your skin feel wonderful are chemicals known as "-cones," such as dimethicone and cyclomethicone. These act like a plastic film by filling in your lines, wrinkles, and pores in order to create a smooth, soft surface. It is hard to feel your skin after using such a product and not be astounded by the texture. But ingredients such as -cones suffocate your skin and prevent it from detoxifying. They also clog your pores, which makes the natural oil in your skin go rancid. Even if you wash the surface of your skin every day, doing so will not clean your pores. Rancid oils break down the collagen in your skin and accelerate aging. Sorry, but they're not miracle workers.

Natural creams work by supplying your skin with moisture that mimics sebum (your skin's natural oil). This allows for complete absorption and will not result in clogged pores. They also rely on active ingredients that allow your skin to repair itself, making it stronger and restoring its natural functions.

Here is an ingredient list for a face cream that illustrates things to avoid:

- aqua (water, green tea [*Camellia sinensis*] leaf aqueous infusion)
- glyceryl polymethacrylate
- glycerin

- ethylene/acrylic acid copolymer
- hydroxypropyl cyclodextrin
- caffeine
- collagen
- gingko (*Gingko biloba*) leaf extract
- grape (*Vitis vinifera*) seed extract
- green tea (*Camellia sinensis*) leaf extract
- European beech (*Fagus sylvatica*) extract
- panthenol
- sorbitol
- tocopherol (vitamin E) acetate
- tocopherol (vitamin E)
- propylene glycol
- bisabolol
- retinol palmitate
- escin
- peanut (*Arachis hypogaea*) oil
- isopropyl myristate
- lecithin
- polyvinyl pyrrolidone (PVP)
- PEG-40
- hydrogenated castor (*Ricinus communis*) bean oil
- allantoin
- sodium carbomer
- alcohol
- triethanolamine
- disodium EDTA
- benzyl alcohol
- methylparaben
- propylparaben
- perfume (fragrance with lemon, nutmeg, orange essential oils)

Contrast this with an ingredient list for a face cream containing helpful ingredients to look for:

- water
- emulsifying wax
- stearic acid
- olive (*Olea europaea*) oil
- organic aloe (*Aloe barbadensis*) leaf juice
- retinol (vitamin A)
- tetrahexyldecyl ascorbate (vitamin C ester)

- wolfberry (*Lycium barbarum*)
- shiitake mushroom (*Lentinus edodes*)
- bamboo (*Bambusa* sp.)
- pomegranate (*Punica granatum*)
- rooibos (*Aspalathus linearis*)
- hibiscus (*Hibiscus sabdariffa*)
- asafetida (*Ferula foetida*)
- pear (*Pyrus communis*)
- white, black, and green teas (*Camellia sinensis*)
- Himalayan raspberry root (*Rubus idaeus*)
- seaweed (*Fucus vesiculosis*)
- lecithin
- carrot (*Daucus carota sativa*) seed oil
- alpha-lipoic acid
- methylsulfonylmethane (MSM)
- wheat (*Triticum vulgare*) amino acids
- oat (*Avena sativa*) amino acids
- tocopherol (vitamin E)
- zinc oxide
- neem (*Melia azadirachta*) seed oil
- rosemary (*Rosmarinus officinalus*) oil
- black willow (*Salix nigra*) bark extract
- lichen (*Usnea barbata*) extract
- potassium sorbate
- sodium benzoate

Alternative Options for Least Amount of Added Toxins— Face Creams

| GOOD

1. Botanical Skin Works Shea Butter Face and Body Lotion

| BETTER

1. Sophyto Normalising Day Face Moisturizer

2. Best Bath Store Intensive Under Eye Treatment

3. Cranberry Lane Radiance Collagen Face Rest (Night Cream)

| BEST

1. Body Botanicals Jojoba & Primrose Moisturizer

2. Suki Eye Repair Balm

3. Grateful Body 30Plus Nourishment Concentrated Rejuvenating Cream

4. Grateful Body 30Plus Eye Cream

5. Suki Balancing Day Lotion

6. Suki Intensive Brightening Crème

7. Sumbody A–Z Face Cream

8. Sumbody Crème Fraiche Face Cream

9. Sumbody Eternal Face Cream

10. Sumbody Delight and DelightFULL Face Cream

11. Natural Family Botanicals Organic Daily Facial Moisturizer

TIPS

Always use your ring finger for applying eye cream and your ring and middle finger for face cream, as they are your weakest fingers and will put less pressure on delicate skin.

Keep your eye cream in the fridge to combat its tendency to cause eye puffiness.

Use your face cream as makeup remover.

Apply face cream under mineral makeup for a smoother look.

Add some mineral makeup to your eye/face cream to make a tinted moisturizer.

Serums

A face serum serves a different function than a cream. It should be applied before, not in place of, a cream; its goal is not to moisturize but to combat specific skin problems. It may fend off dark patches, wrinkles, large pores, blemishes, or the effects of aging. If well-made and used in the proper combination, serums boost the benefits of your cream. Chemical-based serums work like chemical creams—they produce a feeling, not an actual result. They do not repair or heal anything, since the chemicals they contain actually create the problems they are supposed to fix, and instead make your skin feel as though they have.

Here is an ingredient list for a face serum that illustrates things to avoid:

- water
- licorice (*Glykyrrhiza glabra*) root extract
- willowherb (*Epilobium angustifolium*) extract
- grape (*Vitis vinifera*) seed extract
- butylene glycol
- xanthan gum
- tetrasodium EDTA
- methylsilanol ascorbate
- butylene glycol
- SD alcohol 40-B
- methylparaben
- ethylparaben
- diazolidinyl urea
- cucumber (*Cucumis sativus*) extract

Contrast this with an ingredient list for a serum containing helpful ingredients to look for:

- rose hydrosol
- blue green algae (*Aphanizomenon flos-aquae*) extract
- spirulina (*Arthrospira* sp.) extract
- sea parsley (*Palmaria palmata*) extract
- neem (*Melia azadirachta*) seed oil
- black willow (*Salix nigra*) bark extract
- lichen (*Usnea barbata*) extract
- potassium sorbate
- sodium benzoate

Alternative Options for Least Amount of Added Toxins— Serums

Since there are so many "Better" and "Best" options, I decided not to include a "Good" list.

BETTER

1. Super Salve Company VitaNutrient Intensive Vitamin C Treatment

2. Super Salve Company Daily Renewal Peel

BEST

1. Suki Pure Facial Moisture—Nourishing
2. Suki Pure Facial Moisture—Balancing
3. Sumbody Lighten Up Face Serum
4. Sumbody It's About Time Facial Serum
5. Sumbody It's About Time Eye Serum
6. Sumbody Insightful Eye Serum
7. Sumbody Full Infusion Face Serum
8. Sumbody Skin Tight Face Serum
9. Sumbody Eye Believe Serum
10. GeoGrafx Purifying Day Serum
11. GeoGrafx Purifying Night Serum
12. GeoGrafx Normalizing Day Serum
13. GeoGrafx Normalizing Night Serum

TIPS

Choose one serum at a time to combat your specific problem. Switch serums only when the problem has disappeared. Do not use serums unless you have specific issues such as acne, sagging skin, discoloration, dark circles, age issues such as slower cellular turnover, wrinkles, lines, and excessive dryness, or for protection from pollution.

Apply in small, circular, upward motion for better penetration.

Face Oils

Face oils are a relatively new concept to most consumers. We are accustomed to slathering rich creams and lotions on our face, but the truth is, most creams and lotions cannot be metabolized or utilized by the skin on the face. From the neck up, skin needs thinner substances, such as oils, for proper absorption of both the moisture and active ingredients. This is a hard notion for most consumers to swallow, so few major brands make oil-based face moisturizer. The other issue with face oils is that they don't form a good base for makeup. For those who wear makeup daily, face oil is best worn at night. You can also apply a layer of face oil first, wait one minute, and then apply face cream.

It is important for people with oily skin to understand that oil on oil actually negates oil. If you do not apply oil, it sends a message to your skin that you need more oil, and this, in turn, causes your pores to overproduce oil. A well-made face oil will stop this overproduction.

Not all face oils are beneficial. Look for products made with a combination of oils. You want oils that do not clog pores, such as jojoba, olive, and safflower, and oils that help maintain healthy skin, like carrot and rose hip, which contain vitamins A and C.

Here is an ingredient list for a face oil that illustrates things to avoid:

- water
- polysorbate-20
- mineral oil
- jojoba (*Simmondsia chinensis*) seed oil
- olive (*Olea europaea*) leaf extract
- dimethicone
- methylparaben
- ethylparaben
- fragrance

Contrast this with an ingredient list for a face oil containing helpful ingredients to look for:

- pistachio (*Pistacia vera*) oil
- safflower (*Carthamus tinctorius*) seed oil
- apricot (*Prunus armeniaca*) oil
- jojoba (*Simmondsia chinensis*) seed oil
- avocado (*Persea gratissima*) oil
- rose-hip (*Rosa canina*) oil
- camellia (*Camellia sinensis*) oil
- carrot (*Daucus carota sativa*) oil
- grapefruit (*Citrus paradisi*) seed extract

Alternative Options for Least Amount of Added Toxins— Face Oils

| BEST

1. Weleda Almond Facial Oil

2. In Fiore Face Oil Concentré: Calme, Nourrit, Pur

3. Sumbody SumFormula Facial Serum: Normal to Dry Skin, Normal to Oily Skin, Sensitive Skin

4. Lodestar Essentials Chilean Rose Hip Oil

5. Lodestar Essentials Egyptian Wild Carrot Seed Oil

6. Lodestar Essentials Tamanau Oil

7. Natural Family Botanicals Replenishing Facial Oil

8. Flower Peddler Meadow Rose Luxury Facial Oil

TIPS

Face oil can double as an effective makeup remover, but don't use it under makeup.

For intense moisture repair, use oil at night, and seal with a cream.

Chapter 14

Exfoliants

It is better to be beautiful
than to be good,
but it is better to be good
than to be ugly.

— OSCAR WILDE

Once a spa-time fantasy for the fortunate few, now accessible everyday products, exfoliating agents are among the most popular personal-care products in today's market. From our desire for fresher and more vibrant skin came a product aimed at removing dead skin cells and leaving the skin soft, smooth, and beautiful.

Exfoliation is important because it helps combat the visible effects of aging. Many women exclaim with jealousy that men age much more gracefully than women. One reason for this is that many men shave on a regular basis, which exfoliates their faces. In my stores we conduct a demonstration that involves placing Scotch tape on a customer's hand and removing it to illustrate the amount of dead skin lying on the surface of the skin and creating a barrier that is difficult for nutrients to penetrate. This layer of dead skin cells can mix with your skin's oils and create blackheads. While your skin naturally rids itself of the uppermost layers, it needs a hand in making sure they come off completely and at the right time.

There are a few rules that will guide you in the process of exfoliating. The skin underneath your eyes is the most sensitive skin on your face, and you should avoid exfoliating around it. Your entire face is relatively delicate, so you should use a gentler exfoliant on your face than you use on your body. If you have chronic acne, you should consult a dermatologist before exfoliating with anything but a product that eats away your dead skin, because if the acne is bacterial or viral, using a granular substance risks spreading pimples. For everyone, removing dead skin reveals the soft, youthfully vibrant new skin and allows it to absorb nutrients and moisture.

Exfoliating mediums abound. The main natural ones include salt, sugar, walnut shells, apricot kernels, jojoba beads, bamboo, and rice. Basically, they all serve the same purpose but vary in efficacy. Some are too harsh or not harsh enough to remove the proper amount of dead skin cells, and some contain properties that are beneficial for your skin. Any one of these can be suspended in a number of liquids, including oils, milks, and chemical milk shakes.

In addition to these products, some people employ sponges to slough off their dead skin. There is some concern about using natural sponges, because historically they were not harvested in a sustainable manner. However, you can now find farm-raised sponges that have been sustainably harvested. One problem with both natural and synthetic sponges is that if you do not replace them often enough, they can harbor bacteria and mold, which can rub off on your body. Like exfoliants, sponges come in varying degrees of aggressiveness. Sponges do not provide any additional benefits, such as moisture, but if kept out of stagnant water and replaced often, they are effective exfoliating agents. The final types of exfoliating products are ones that don't contain any type of grain, but rather eat away the bacteria.

Chemically concocted exfoliating products pose a unique threat to your health because not only are they designed to be scrubbed on from head to toe, but when they remove the dead skin, they create an inviting pathway for the chemicals to slide in to your bloodstream. Ironically, these chemical-based products accelerate the signs of aging as well as sucking up your skin's natural moisture—exactly what a good exfoliant should prevent. Because of the breadth of exposure to chemicals and their easy access to your bloodstream, exfoliants are important products to replace with a natural alternative. Luckily, these alternatives are fairly easy to come by, and while some can be slightly more expensive than the chemical versions, the extra cost is mitigated by a decreased need for additional moisturizing.

Body Scrubs

Salt and sugar form the base for the most common body scrubs, but other exfoliating agents include granulated grape seed and ground-up loofah, which got their launch as a popular treatments at spas. The increasing availability of these products has made them accessible to everyone. Oil-free scrubs are rare, and most conventional products are a chemical soup of ingredients that make your skin feel exfoliated, moisturized, and smooth. Common substitutes for oil include glycerin, a derivative of animal and/or vegetable fat; mineral oil, a derivative of petroleum; or numerous combinations of chemicals that "feel" like and give the consistency of oil. These ingredients dehydrate your skin and require the use of additional moisturizers. While there are some products, like shampoo, in which chemicals add desirable qualities such as lather or consistency, scrubs are not one of them. Scrubs are more effective and feel better when they are made of natural ingredients. Chemicals are used in scrubs to create a thicker texture, a smoother feel, a stronger scent, and as filler (chemical fillers are far less expensive than natural ingredients and reduce the cost of making the product). You can achieve all the same effects and much more benefit by using a natural product. However, without the inexpensive fillers and chemicals, they may cost a little bit more. Interestingly enough, quite often it is the better products that cost less. In a drugstore, the chemical counterparts generally cost less, but in boutiques, spas, and department stores they are usually more expensive than the natural products. So look for the best value on the cleanest product with the best benefits when you are shopping.

The common unnecessary ingredients to look for in scrubs are fragrance, artificial colors, preservatives, and petroleum products. Because oils go rancid naturally (just like the oils you use to cook with, when left in your cupboard they will go bad over time), some companies use chemical preservatives to extend shelf life and prevent them from spoiling. Natural preservation methods for oils are available, such as salt; a product using natural preservation should come with the date it was bottled, so you know how long it will last. The sole reason for choosing mineral oil over avocado oil or making any other quality sacrifice is cost and shelf life. The longer the shelf life, the longer the product you are buying has been sitting. It is quite common for chemical products to sit years before they reach the shelf. It is true the oils would be rancid in a naturally preserved product if they were left this long on back shelves. Companies producing "natural" products must "turn" their products much faster. So this means that once again it is harder for natural companies to make a profit, but at least you, as the consumer, are getting a fresher product. At Sumbody, we aim to have all our products on our store shelves within one month of them being manufactured. Then, we add another month to turn at the store shelf. This means your product is still fresh and active and has a long shelf life remaining after you purchase it. I am always asked how long a natural product will stay preserved. This differs, depending on the product, but it is usually between one to two years. One to two years is more then enough time to finish a 1 oz container of face cream or a 4 oz container of a face cleanser. If you have not used your products in that time, throw them away. No amount of preservation would help, I tell people if they haven't used it, it probably was not a good purchase to begin with. If you had liked it, it would have been gone.

One of the issues with extended preservation is the amount of time a product can sit on a shelf or in a warehouse before you purchase it. While sitting on the shelf, all the active ingredients are losing their potency, and by the time you use them, they are not as active, or potent, as they were originally.

The greatest challenge in formulating a natural scrub is suspending the oil and preventing separation. Products with a layer of oil on the top tend to be more wasteful because you lose a disproportionate amount of oil through drips and spills and can find yourself left with a base of dry salt or sugar. Well-suspended scrubs are also easier to use. When you shop for a scrub, look for one with butters; your body needs the richer butters to provide the proper moisture from the neck down, and it thrives on rich moisture (of course, you also have to consider your body and personal preferences). Most people are hesitant to use salt scrubs because they think of salt as a drying agent. However, if the salt scrub is formulated correctly, it will replenish your body's moisture as well as any other scrub. Shaving is something else to consider when choosing between salt and sugar. If used after shaving, salt can sting and cause redness, just like going into the ocean with an open cut, whereas sugar will not. Both are fine to use before shaving.

Just as many consumers believe salt is a drying agent, they believe sugar doesn't do enough as an exfoliant because it doesn't feel as abrasive as salt. While it is true that sugar feels softer, that doesn't mean it is not an effective scrub. Glycolic acid, a natural compound found in sugar, helps eat away your dead skin cells. You should avoid sugar scrubs if you have any type of yeast rash on your body, because the sugar will feed the yeast and worsen the rash.

One concern with both salt and sugar scrubs is microabrasions. Both sugar and salt are composed of cubic granules, which can have sharp edges, but because of the way they are used, this does not pose a threat to your skin. Both salt and sugar dissolve in water, so as soon as you begin applying a scrub in the bath or shower, the substance mixes with water from your body and bath, immediately beginning to dissolve the square particles into circles. This process will take longer with a larger granule, so if you are using a large-granule scrub, be sure to use plenty of water and scrub slowly, using a circular motion.

The last question on the table is whether to splurge on a more expensive, often more enticing-sounding scrub that incorporates loofah, grape seed, or any other exfoliating granule. The truth is, salt and sugar do such a great job and give you all the moisture you need. So in this case, it is not worth spending the extra money for what is often an equal or substandard product. Some of the beneficial ingredients you should look for in a scrub are pure oils, such as avocado, apricot, and sunflower, butters such as shea or mango, and pure essential oils.

With a scrub, you won't have to adjust to anything by making the switch to natural—and you might well be amazed at the results!

Here is an ingredient list for a salt scrub that illustrates things to avoid:

- isopropyl palmitate
- beeswax (*Cera alba*)
- sucrose
- laureth-4
- silicon oxide
- fragrance
- shea (*Butyrospermum parkii*) butter extract
- steareth-21
- borage (*Borago officinalis*) seed oil
- wheat germ (*Triticum vulgare*) oil
- mineral oil
- tocopherol (vitamin E) acetate
- jojoba (*Simmondsia chinensis*) seed oil
- sesame (*Sesamum indicum*)
- avocado (*Persea gratissima*) oil
- t-butylhydroquinone (TBHQ)
- glyceryl oleate

Contrast this with an ingredient list for a scrub containing helpful ingredients to look for:

- pure Pacific sea salt
- safflower (*Carthamus tinctorius*) seed oil
- jojoba (*Simmondsia chinensis*) seed oil
- shea (*Butyrospermum parkii*) butter
- green tea (*Camellia sinensis*) extract (extracted in safflower oil)
- pure essential oil blend

Alternative Options for Least Amount of Added Toxins— Body Scrubs and Face Scrubs

GOOD

1. Alba Sugar Cane Body Polish
2. Sunshine Spa Vanilla Orange Brown Sugar Scrub

BETTER

1. ABRA Therapeutic Peppermint & Oats Skin Refining Scrub
2. Zosimos Botanicals Sugar Scrub
3. Sumbody Sugar Scrub: Get Lei'd, Sex on the Beach, Coconut & Cream, Milky Rich, Wishes
4. Sumbody Salt Scrub: Get Lei'd, Sex on the Beach, Coconut & Cream, Milky Rich, Wishes

BEST

1. ABRA Therapeutic Green Tea Body Scrub
2. Zosimos Botanicals Salt Scrub
3. Lunaroma Coffee Body Scrub
4. Lunaroma Salt Glow
5. Lunaroma Sugar Body Polish
6. Hugo Natural Botanical Apothecary French Lavender Dead Sea Salt Body Scrub
7. Hugo Natural Botanical Apothecary Brown Sugar & Kumquat Body Scrubs
8. Sumbody Sugar Scrub: Citrus Splash, Lavender Wave, Mint, Satsuma Cardamom

9. Sumbody Salt Scrub: Citrus Splash, Lavender Wave, Mint, Satsuma Cardamom, California Sunshine

TIPS

Use a salt or sugar scrub first, then shave. The exfoliation results in a closer, smoother shave. Salt scrubs will slightly sting in open wounds, nicks, or cuts, so you may prefer to use a sugar scrub.

Keep scrub by the sink to use after washing; it will help keep your hands soft and moisturized.

Use soap before you scrub and do not soap your body off afterward. Let the water gently rinse off the salt or sugar and then pat dry.

Face Scrubs

The skin on our face is extremely delicate and requires special care while scrubbing. You should always use your ring and middle fingers, because they are the weakest (and therefore the most kind to delicate skin), and scrub in a gentle upward circular motion. One of the first popular face scrubs sold used crushed apricot kernels as its exfoliating agent. Think of crushing an apricot kernel. It shatters into small, sharp, jagged fragments, which cause microabrasions on your face. These small cuts and tears damage your skin and accelerate aging. Stay away from face scrubs that contain an exfoliating agent that does not dissolve. Look for something dissolvable or any type of spherical granule, such as jojoba beads, and powders, such as almond or rice. While these powders are not dissolvable, they become mushy when mixed with water and are soft enough that they will not cause damage. Unfortunately, apricot and walnut kernels are hot trends on the market. If you just "have" to use them, compromise with finely powdered apricot or walnut instead of using the crushed matter. It is not the greatest solution, but it will allow you to avoid some of the damage.

Not only are there a number of exfoliating agents to choose from, but face scrubs are manufactured in a variety of bases. Most are suspended in creams, and some contain glycolic or alpha hydroxy acids, which eat away dead skin. These acids are a different way of exfoliating, and if you are using this type of scrub, you should know your product thoroughly. First, be aware that many people have allergies to these acids. Second, while many effective acids, including many fruit acids, are natural, there is also a plethora of synthetic acids that are not as good for your skin. A high percentage of these will harm your skin, while a low percentage will not remove enough of your dead skin.

Chemical face scrubs that use synthetic acids tend to make skin age faster over time. They can also leave your face red, raw, and irritated. Chemicals can give you faster results in the short run but cause a host of issues in the long run. Some people choose the short-term effects that are provided by chemicals, not knowing or caring about the future havoc the product will wreak on their skin. As a culture, we tend to live in the moment, not thinking about consequences. We want immediate results and we are not always willing to be patient. If you insist on using your chemical peel, I suggest you do a patch test. Take a dime-sized amount and place it on your inner wrist before purchasing the product to see if you will react negatively. Never do a chemical peel before a special event, just in case you have a reaction.

Here is an ingredient list for a face scrub that illustrates things to avoid:

- water
- amara (*Citrus aurantium*) flower water
- butylene glycol
- lecithin
- bethenyl betaine
- glycerin
- polysorbate-60
- propylene glycol stearate
- polysorbate-20
- sorbitan laurate
- polysorbate-80
- sodium chloride
- papaya (*Carica papaya*) extract
- buchu (*Barosma betulina*) leaf oil
- grapefruit (*Citrus paradisi*) peel oil
- eucalyptus (*Eucalyptus globulus*) leaf oil
- Siberian fir (*Abies sibirica*) oil

- arvensis leaf oil
- bitter almond (*Prunus amygdalus amara*) kernel oil
- limonene
- apricot (*Prunus armeniaca*)
- walnut (*Juglans regia*) shell powder
- carnauba (*Copernicia cerifera*) wax
- mango (*Mangifera indica*) extract
- propylene glycol laurate
- papain
- carbomer
- phosphorate phosphate
- dimethyl isosorbide
- potassium sorbate
- sodium dehydroacetate
- tetrasodium EDTA
- phenoxyethanol
- methylparaben
- ethylparaben
- propylparaben
- butylparaben
- isopropylparaben
- isobutylparaben
- essential oil

Contrast this with an ingredient list for a face scrub containing helpful ingredients to look for:

- aloe (*Aloe barbadensis*) leaf juice
- German chamomile (*Matricaria recutita*) flower
- water
- jojoba (*Simmondsia chinensis*) seed oil
- emulsifying wax
- kosher vegetable glycerin
- evening primrose (*Oenothera biennis*) oil
- rose hip seed (*Rosa canina*) oil
- palm stearic acid
- shea (*Butyrospermum parkii*) butter
- vitamin E
- lecithin
- neem (*Melia azadirachta*) seed oil
- sodium bicarbonate

- xanthan gum
- jojoba (*Simmondsia chinensis*) wax beads
- nettle (*Urtica dioica*) leaf extracted in jojoba oil
- birch bark (*Betula pubescens*) extracted in jojoba oil
- orrisroot (*Iris germanica*) extracted in jojoba oil
- burdock (*Arctium lappa*) extracted in jojoba oil
- rosemary (*Rosmarinus officinalis*) leaf extracted in jojoba oil

Alternative Options for Least Amount of Added Toxins— Face Scrubs

Since face scrubs are used by many people interchangeably with face cleansers, face scrubs have been included in the "Good," "Better," "Best" list for face cleansers on page 177 in the next chapter.

TIPS

Use almond meal for a simple but effective face scrub and lip exfoliant.

For enhanced results, use your face scrub in the shower. Your skin will be wet, pores will be open, and dead skin will be easier to remove.

Chapter 15

Face Cleansers, Toners, and Masks

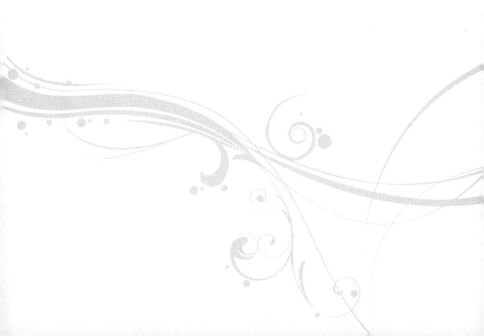

The skin on our face is extremely delicate and sensitive, and it is exposed to the elements on a daily basis. Our face is also our first point of encounter with the world, so we tend to be the most concerned with its appearance. When we speak of someone as beautiful, pretty, or handsome, we are usually referring to that person's face. It is no wonder that consumers want to find the very best products to help them maintain their beauty and youthful appearance. Cleansing regularly is a necessity; it removes dirt and can loosen stagnant oils from pores, helps combat acne, and slows the signs of aging such as wrinkles and fine lines.

Cleansers come in many forms, including creams, milks, foams, oils, gels, and bars. One of the most important aspects of a good face cleanser is that it maintains the skin's pH level. The skin on your face is fairly acidic, with a pH of about 5.5, which helps rid it of bacteria and fungus. Bar soaps, even handmade ones, throw off your skin's pH, since they are very astringent and remove the acid mantle, leaving your skin exposed. There are some bar soaps that are marketed specifically to balance your skin's pH, but I have tested many of them and found that they fall short. Creams, milks, foams, oils, and gels have the potential to be good or bad in terms of pH. To find out where your cleanser stands, go to your local pool-supply company or possibly your drugstore and buy pH strips to test your product. Your cleanser should fall within the range of about 4.2 and 5.6.

There are many other issues that dictate which cleanser is right for your skin. However, just because you have oily skin does not mean you should stay away from a cream cleanser or a face moisturizer. In fact, by not applying enough moisture to your face, you're causing your skin to overproduce oil.

Unfortunately, you really have to scour the shelves to find natural cleansers. Most are chemical cocktails filled with lathering agents such as sodium lauryl sulfate, PEGs, and many other chemicals. Many contain only one natural ingredient—water. While chemical cleansers can clean your skin, they cause myriad other problems, such as dryness, wrinkles, and redness during the cleaning process.

The following are important steps to follow when washing your face:

1. Wash your hands thoroughly at the start and remove all makeup to avoid rubbing dirt and bacteria into your skin.

2. Moisten your face with warm water. Avoid hot water, as it strips your face of its natural oils and moisture.

3. Massage the cleanser into your skin using your ring and middle fingers in an upward circular motion to open your pores. Avoid massaging the delicate skin directly beneath your eyes. Leave the cleanser on for one to two minutes to loosen the dirt. If you insist on using soap, rinse it off immediately.

4. Rinse your face with water or a soft washcloth, and pat dry.

5. Be sure to follow these four steps on your neck as well as your face.

Here is an ingredient list for a face cleanser that illustrates things to avoid:

- water
- glycerin
- cetyl alcohol
- stearic acid
- PPG-15 stearyl ether
- palmitic acid
- steareth-21
- methyl gluceth-20
- polysorbate-60
- triethanolamine (TEA)
- perfume
- grapefruit (*Citrus paradisi*) extract
- panthenol
- tocopheryl acetate
- peppermint (*Mentha piperita*) leaf extract
- T-butyl alcohol
- ammonium polyacryloyldimethyl taurate
- disodium EDTA
- myristic acid

- myristyl alcohol
- stearyl alcohol
- propylparaben
- phenoxyethanol
- imidazolidinyl urea
- methylparaben
- benzyl salicylate
- limonene
- geraniol
- linolool

Contrast this with an ingredient list for a face cleanser containing helpful ingredients to look for:

- sage (*Salvia officinalis*), thyme (*Thymus vulgaris*), and rosemary (*Rosmarinus officinalis*) infusions
- sunflower (*Helianthus annuus*) oil
- grape seed (*Vitis vinifera*) oil
- lavender (*Lavandula angustifolia*) extract
- rosemary (*Rosmarinus officinalis*) extract
- 100% natural beeswax (*Cera alba*)
- pure vegetable glycerin
- fair-trade cocoa (*Theobroma cacao*) butter
- honeysuckle (*Lonicera japonica*) extract
- kaolin
- organic oat (*Avena sativa*) milk
- lemon (*Citrus medica limonum*) oil
- non-GMO lecithin
- cetearyl alcohol
- food-grade xanthan and arabic gums
- aroma (pure premium steam-distilled essential oil)

Alternative Options for Least Amount of Added Toxins— Face Cleansers

Since face cleansers and scrubs are used by many people interchangeably, recommendations for face scrubs, which were discussed in the previous chapter, are included here.

GOOD

1. Burt's Bees Orange Essence Facial Cleanser
2. Sophyto Deep Pore Foaming Cleanser

3. Kiss My Face Obsessively Organic Start Up Exfoliating Face Wash

4. Alaffia Rooibos & Shea Butter Antioxidant Facial Cleanser

BETTER

1. Shebas Secrets Face of Beauty Herbal Scrub

2. Shebas Secrets Face of Beauty Nourishing Scrub

BEST

1. Natural Family Botanicals Lavender Clay Facial Scrub

2. Weleda Almond Cleansing Lotion

3. In Fiore Treate Gentle Cleansing Base

4. Dr. Hauschka Cleansing Milk

5. Dr. Hauschka Cleansing Cream

6. Pangea Organics Egyptian Calendula & Blood Orange Facial Cleanser

7. Jasco Organics Renew Exfoliating Cleanser

8. Botanical Skin Works Soothing Oats Facial Cleanser

9. Suki Moisture-Rich Cleansing Lotion

10. Suki Exfoliating Foaming Cleanser

11. Lush Angels on Bare Skin Cleanser

12. Lush Herbalism Cleanser

13. Sumbody C Me Glow Face Cleanser

14. Sumbody Coal Train Charcoal Cleanser

15. Sumbody Go Jojo Facial Cleanser

16. Sumbody Polishing Grains

17. Sumbody Manna Face Cleanser

18. Sumbody Bee Delighted Facial Scrub

> **TIP** Try a nonfoaming cleanser for one month to see if you can adjust and live without foam. This way you'll be avoiding some of the worst chemicals found in face cleansers. Additionally, although you may like foam, it is not the element that does the cleaning.

Toners

One of the most important steps in cleansing is toning. When I first started working with skin, I used to say, "Save your money; if there's one step to skip, it's toner." Now I totally disagree. If you are taking the time to cleanse and are spending money on good moisturizers, serums, masks, and natural cleansers, you have to tone. Otherwise, you are leaving your pores open and subject to the dirt, oils, smog, and grime of everyday life. Toner restores your skin's natural pH, gets rid of the last bit of dirt and oil, closes pores, and gets skin ready for the day. Many toners also contain active ingredients that help reduce inflammation, decrease wrinkles, and get rid of dead skin cells. It is sort of like exercising your pores. Opening and closing your pores pushes the gunk out. Sometimes I suggest people put toner in the refrigerator, rinse their face with warm water, pat dry, and then apply their toner. The warm water opens their pores and the cold toner closes them. This pushes out the dirt and stagnant oils in your pores and keeps your pores in shape. You can repeat this process several times before applying serum or moisturizer.

Here is an ingredient list for a toner that illustrates things to avoid:

- botanical infusion of clary sage (*Salvia sclarea*) and chamomile
- polysorbate-20
- aloe (*Aloe barbadensis*) gel
- red raspberry extract
- blackberry extract
- alfalfa extract
- artichoke extract
- glycerin
- sodium PCA
- hydrolyzed glycosaminoglycans
- panthenol
- allantoin
- dimethylaminoethanol (DMAE)
- retinol palmitate
- tocopherol (vitamin E) acetate
- phenoxyethanol
- propylparaben
- methylparaben

- French lavender (*Lavandula angustifolia*) essential oil
- rosewood essential oil
- Roman chamomile (*Anthemis nobilis*) essential oil

Contrast this with an ingredient list for a toner containing helpful ingredients to look for:

- water
- alcohol
- witch hazel (*Hamamelis virginiana*)
- lemon (*Citrus medica limonum*)
- bearded iris (*Iris germanica*)
- fragrance (from natural essential oils)
- linalool (from natural essential oils)
- citronellal (from natural essential oils)
- geraniol (from natural essential oils)

Alternative Options for Least Amount of Added Toxins— Toners

GOOD

1. Better Botanicals Juniper Toning Mist
2. Best Bath Store Pore Refining Facial Toner
3. Organic Apoteke Balancing Rose Toner

BETTER

1. In Fiore Vitale Toning Floral Essence
2. Alaffia Rooibos & Shea Antioxidant Facial Toner
3. Sumbody It's About Time Toner

BEST

1. Weleda Iris Facial Toner
2. Dr. Hauschka Clarifying Toner
3. Dr. Hauschka Rhythmic Conditioner, Sensitive
4. Dr. Hauschka Rhythmic Night Conditioner
5. Grateful Body Daily Facial Toner
6. Grateful Body 30Plus Spot Toner
7. Suki Facial Toner

8. Grateful Body Environmental Impact Facial Toner

9. Sumbody Get Closure Acne Toner

10. Sumbody Facial Toner: Cucumber, Rose, Neroli

TIPS

During the summer, keep your toner in the fridge to help cool your face and close your pores.

Make "ice cubes" with your toner and use under your eyes to decrease puffiness.

Masks

Masks can do just about anything from hydrating to removing blemishes caused by acne to just making your face glow. When you see how many properties masks can have, you'll realize that they are one of the real workhorses of face care.

There are three main types of masks; deep pore masks, mid pore masks, and specific-issue masks. Deep pore cleansers break up the oils and dirt in your pores and pull them out so your pores can function properly. While many labels and salespeople will disagree, for most people once a month is frequent enough for deep cleansing. The only reason you will hear differently is if someone is trying to "sell you, not tell you." However, your masks should fit your lifestyle. If you play sports, travel a lot, commute, or live in a smoggy city, you will need to bump up your frequency to two to four times a month so you can purge all of the dirt, smog, and stagnant oil building up in your pores. Dust, pollution, car exhaust, and oils mix together in your pores and create a plug that nutrients and topical products cannot penetrate. Deep pore cleansers are the most important masks because they strip your pores and clean them out so your skin can breathe and function properly. If you have dry skin, deep pore cleansers allow the moisture to penetrate your pores instead of sitting uselessly on the surface of your face. If you have oily skin, clogged pores block your skin's natural oils from reaching the surface and trigger your skin to produce more oil. This starts a vicious cycle of overproducing and creating excess oil to combat what the skin perceives as a lack of moisture. If you are using serums and creams to combat unwanted conditions and to nourish your skin, masks allow these products to penetrate the skin so they can work, as opposed to just laying on the surface.

The second type of mask is the mid pore cleanser. These masks should be applied once a week, on average, but again this depends on your lifestyle. These masks can contain ingredients, such as alpha hydroxy, that help with issues, such as increasing the skin's elasticity, getting rid of dead skin cells, and reversing signs of aging, and claim to clean the mid pores and provide an acid peel. These ingredients are not necessary or beneficial for a mid pore cleaner and will cost you more without giving you the results you are looking for. Mid pore cleaning masks are meant solely to keep the mid pore clean in between the deep pore cleaning and feed the skin with vitamins and nutrients in the process. These types of masks help maintain healthy, vibrant skin. It is best to buy a mask that is designed to tackle specific problems: A mask that tries to "take on" too many skin issues can be ineffective overall.

Not as intense as deep pore cleanses, these keep your pores clean in between deep cleanses. Each month we try to do a deep cleaning in our home, which means scrubbing toilets, cleaning stove grilles, washing windows, and pushing out accumulated muck and grime. Every week we try to maintain the cleanliness by washing dishes, putting our things away, making our beds, and doing the laundry. Deep pore cleansers are like scrubbing the bathroom tiles, while mid pore cleansers are more like folding the laundry.

The third type of mask has nothing to do with cleaning, but rather is formulated to combat innumerable skin grievances. These masks rehydrate skin that has lost moisture as it ages, balance pH, brighten dullness, fade age spots and discoloration, and reduce wrinkles to restore a vibrant, healthy, youthful glow to your face.

In conjunction with the rest of your skin-care regime, masks can give your skin a boost. Gone are the days of feeling the burn of a drying mask as it crumbles and creases on your face. You can "hydrolyze your mask on" by placing a warm, damp hand towel over your face, leaving your mouth and nose uncovered. This technique keeps the mask moist and open pores. Water and steam help the mask achieve deeper penetration and create a more thorough, lasting effect.

Many people exclaim that they are too busy for masks, but the five to fifteen minutes using a mask takes from your day can add years to the quality and appearance of your skin. If you're a holdout who insists you don't have time, I'm taking away your last excuse. You can apply a mask in the shower. Everyone takes a shower, and it is the perfect time for a mask. The natural steam in the shower will hydrolyze the mask on for you. For maximum results, wash your face and put your mask on first thing when you get in, and rinse just before you exit.

Here is an ingredient list for a mask that illustrates things to avoid:

- water
- algae extract
- wheat (*Triticum vulgare*) protein
- PEG-32
- polyvinyl pyrrolidone (PVP)
- hydrolyzed lupine protein
- PPG-1-PEG-9 lauryl glycol ether
- comfrey (*Symphytum officinale*) leaf extract
- polysorbate-80
- cetyl acetate
- acetylated lanolin alcohol
- carbomer
- tromethamine
- pyridoxine hydrochloride (vitamin B-6)
- panthenol
- tetrasodium EDTA
- propylene glycol
- fragrance
- phenoxyethanol
- methylparaben
- butylparaben
- ethylparaben
- propylparaben
- isobutylparaben
- FD&C Red 4

Contrast this with an ingredient list for a mask containing helpful ingredients to look for:

- organic, ethically wildcrafted, or biodynamically grown extracts (in pure grain alcohol) of green tea (*Camellia sinensis*), nori, cucumber, parsley, green papaya, and pineapple
- organic golden jojoba (*Simmondsia chinensis*) seed oil
- organic safflower (*Carthamus tinctorius*) seed oil
- organic avocado (*Persea americana*) oil
- organic aloe (*Aloe barbadensis*) gel
- organic or biodynamically grown herbal infusions in jojoba (*Simmondsia chinensis*) oil of sage (*Salvia officinalis*), red clover (*Trifolium pratense*) blossoms, horsetail (*Equisetum arvense*), and comfrey (*Symphytum officinale*) root
- organic raw honey
- organic black cumin seed oil
- organic hydrosols of rose (*Rosa canina*) and lavender (*Lavandula angustifolia*)
- cayenne
- olive squalene oil
- soy lecithin
- organic sage (*Salvia officinalis*) and rosemary (*Rosmarinus officinalis*) antioxidants
- grapefruit (*Citris paradisi*) seed extract
- vitamins A, C, and E

Alternative Options for Least Amount of Added Toxins— Masks

GOOD

1. Shebas Secrets French Clay Facial Mask

BETTER

1. Eco-Beauty Organics Facial Peeling: Soft, Strong
2. Shebas Secrets Coconut Milk by the Sea Facial Mask
3. Cranberry Lane Firming Face Hydrator Mask
4. Cranberry Lane Clarifying Acne Mask

BEST

1. Natural Family Botanicals Restorative Herbal Clay Mask
2. Shebas Secrets Farm & Sea Facial Mask

3. Best Bath Store Dead Sea Mud Mask

4. Jasco Organics Essence Spa Facial

5. Botanical Skin Works Soothing Oats Facial Mask

6. Suki Intensive Brightening Masque

7. Suki Transformative Cleansing Clay

8. Grateful Body 30 Plus Enzyme Mask

9. Best Bath Store Acne Treatment Gel

10. Sumbody Face Mask: Deep Sea, Crème de la Crème, Bee Euphoria, Get Cultured

11. Super Salve Company Green Clay Exfoliant Mask

TIPS

Mix one part apple cider vinegar with six parts water and wash your face with it. Then warm your mask before applying it. The apple cider vinegar helps eat away dead skin cells, promote circulation, restore your skin's pH, and make skin glow.

For better results, wash your face before applying a mask with warm water and cleanser.

PART III

What's a
Busy Woman to Do?

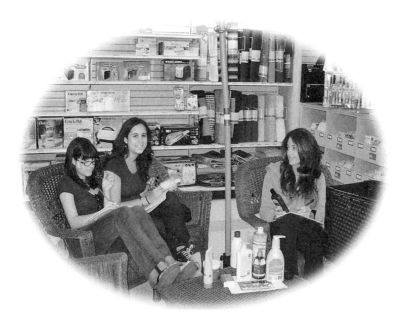

The Burnes gals visit CVS

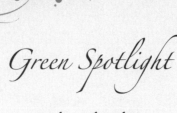

Green Spotlight

Keisha Whitaker,
Model, Entreprenuer, and Activist

"What I find most attractive is confidence. [I am] someone who knows herself, knows what her assets are, and is confident in her own skin. I have three daughters, and I feel it is imperative that we are good examples for our children of how to be healthy and happy in your given body. I teach my children just that, to be happy in their own skin. Not only do I teach them to be happy, but I also teach them how they can do all of this in a responsible way—for themselves and for the planet.

"I work my best assets. It's all about knowing what your assets are and emphasizing them. For me, I choose to work on what I love about myself as opposed to trying to change what I do not. I do not have large breasts, but I would never choose to have breast surgery because of the health concerns associated with it. My daughters look up to me, and I want to let them know this is Mommy's body and this is your body, and everybody's body is different. I want to teach them to be happy in their own skin—they don't need to change it.

"People are becoming aware of the issues of toxins, being green, and doing things to help the planet. Right now it can be overwhelming because we're at the beginning; one day, as we progress generation by generation, it'll be part of our life.

"People want to do something, and little by little we're learning what simple things we can do and changes we can make. I try to eat organic, just started composting, put in eco-friendly air-conditioning, and changed out all the light bulbs to become more energy-efficient.

"I really admire when large companies take it upon themselves to make positive and impactful changes. For instance, Clorox now has a natural green brand, and it is readily available so people are exposed to it regardless of their financial situation; they are able to make a choice. It is imperative that we make these choices accessible to the masses.

"One way we can make positive change for future generations is to be open to change and to seek new knowledge. I am raising my daughters with more awareness than I had when I was growing up. Lucky for us, in this day and age we have choices, more information, and natural alternatives. This is a big change from the way I was raised and what was available to my mom. My house was Pine-Sol clean. My eyes would burn, but the house would smell like what I thought was fresh and squeaky clean. Now I know I was inhaling dangerous chemicals. I didn't know any better because I had never been exposed to anything else.

"When I met my husband, he was very progressive, a vegetarian, into vitamins and health-food stores. We have progressed and grown a lot over the years. My house does not smell Pine-Sol clean; I use natural cleaning products. I am conscious of so many things that I did not even have a concept of before. When we travel and stay in hotels, I have my daughters shower instead of taking a bath. Who knows what chemicals they used to clean; I do not want my children soaking in them. If I do have a choice for something natural in place of something chemical, I will choose the natural alternative. My daughters have been using pure Castile soap forever because I knew that was the natural choice. I am conscious of the dangers associated with drinking out of plastic. I bring my own bags to the grocery store, and I continue to learn more every day. The more I learn, the more I change my habits. I change my habits because I am concerned about the effect of what I am consuming on the environment and my family's health.

"Like my family and me, many people are becoming increasingly aware of the dangers of toxins we are exposed to daily. We know now that living green is necessary for our children's health and that of our planet. We all want to do something, but it can be overwhelming. We do not need to do everything. Little by little we can learn what simple things we can do and what changes we can make. This is why I feel this book is so important and carries such a good message for women. Within these pages you can find the information you need to make the choices that are right for you and your family. Deborah defines the line between what is natural or not, and gives you healthy alternatives. No one's saying you have to be perfect, but if we all do a little bit, we can make a big difference. I deeply appreciate Deborah's knowledge about natural beauty. Most of all, I love having natural alternatives that work!

"As women, we don't need twenty different lotions and fifty different creams to feel beautiful. It goes back to my belief in confidence. If we're putting products on our skin that are natural and good for the planet and have results, we can be confident in our choices and confident in our beauty."

Chapter 16

Chemical-Free
Makeovers

*Consumers believe that
"If it's on the market, it can't hurt me,"
and this belief is sometimes wrong.*

— JOHN BAILEY, PHD, DIRECTOR OF THE FDA'S
OFFICE OF COSMETICS AND COLORS,
FROM AN ARTICLE IN THE
MAY–JUNE 1998 **FDA CONSUMER**

Even for people who aren't concerned about exposure to potentially harmful chemicals, a chemical-free makeover can be appealing. Almost everyone is concerned about their skin's appearance, and eliminating chemicals will work wonders.

The following are ten signs your skin is suffering from chemical overload:

1. dullness or lackluster quality
2. redness, rashes, or irritation
3. excessive dryness, taut feeling, eczema patches
4. itching
5. flaking
6. enlarged pores
7. acne, blackheads, bumps
8. small abrasions and/or zits that take a while to heal
9. oily skin
10. signs of premature aging

These ten signs are some of the most common skin ailments, and they are caused not only by chemicals but also by sun exposure, hormones, and a number of other factors. Chemicals increase and exaggerate these symptoms even though they are originally caused by another factor. If your skin shows significant changes or if you are having problems you haven't had your whole life, you can often look to chemical exposure as the culprit. Even if you've always had eczema, it might have been caused by exposure to chemicals. Chemicals are on our clothing finish, in our detergent, and in many other places where they can seep into our skin and cause irritation. While there are other reasons these signs can occur, you would be surprised by how often altering skin care can easily correct many of these issues. Our bodies were not created to have to combat hundreds of chemicals on a daily basis, and when we remove this added workload, our skin gets a chance to breathe and heal itself.

Beyond changing the products you use, there are other ways to help your skin be beautiful. The following are ten ways to beautify your skin:

1. Drink plenty of water. The first thing your skin loses as it ages is hydration, and you need to hydrate from the inside out.

2. Watch your diet—how you eat shows up on your face first. Reduce alcohol, sugar, and caffeine intake, and don't smoke.

3. Stay out of excessive wind, cold, sun, and dry heat. Wind and cold are dehydrating. When in these elements wear your sunglasses; they protect the eye area, the most delicate and first-to-wrinkle place on your face, from damage.

4. Avoid excessive tanning.

5. Don't wear heavy makeup.

6. Remove all makeup before bed.

7. Do a deep pore cleansing once a month.

8. Be sure to get enough essential fatty acids in your diet.

9. Get plenty of rest. Your skin does most of its repair work at night.

10. Exercise to sweat.

Here are some additional tips for beautiful skin:

◇ Avoid stress and anger. Learn ways you can manage these conditions.

◇ Have fun. Spend time doing what you love.

◇ Have sex.

◇ Make time for family and friends.

It is one thing to read about a situation and another to experience it firsthand. Below are examples of real people and their experience going through the exact process I advocate throughout this book. I chose two people with different skin types and different lifestyles. One is a high-powered executive in the hotel and spa industry; the other is a mother of two on a very tight budget.

When doing a chemical-free makeover, I request that people not change anything else in their lives so they can see how the switch to natural products alone affects their skin and overall health. However, if you are really committed to cleansing your body of toxins, go ahead and change your exercise and dietary habits and cut back on your consumption of alcohol and tobacco. This will allow you to see the full potential of your skin to be vibrant and healthy while you stay away from chemicals and reduce your negative impact on the planet.

The Executive

Tracy is an executive in the hotel and spa industry, and she is committed to providing truly natural products for her customers. She could purchase cheap containers and commercial hotel-grade bulk shampoo but instead is choosing to pay twice as much for the natural alternative. She's backing her commitment with her pocketbook. I have formulated many products for her, and I've offered to cut corners. (At Sumbody I'm a purist, but because these products were for another company I was willing to find some safe synthetics to cut down the cost.) She wanted no part in it. I admire her dedication to providing natural products. It is one thing to advertise all-natural products or to choose mostly all-natural products, but it is quite another to reduce profit for that choice. Most of her customers would not even notice if her products contained chemicals—she makes this choice because her company feels passionately about it.

I compiled a list of all the products Tracy reported using on herself and her one-year-old, along with the full ingredient list for each one. This gave her a chance to see all of the ingredients in one place and assess her overall exposure. Later we will see what she chose to eliminate and assess how much she lowered her overall chemical exposure.

The following are the products Tracy reported using, along with my assessments (notice that she reported using two sunscreens and two types of lip balm—she could cut down her exposure simply by choosing one of each):

1. Encantado Lotion

Right away I noticed that the ingredients were not listed in accordance with the standard format. Also, water is listed twice. This made me wonder why, and what the company might be hiding. This lotion contained two ingredients known to be toxic (dehydroacetic acid, benzyl alcohol) and two questionable ones (sodium PCA, panthenol), as well as several safe synthetics. It also lists several extracts, but we don't know what they are extracted in. This could make a huge difference, as many of the ingredients used for extracting are extremely harmful.

Let's take a closer look:

◇ sodium PCA: Animal studies show endocrine-system disruption and other harmful effects. While it is considered fairly safe, we lack enough scientific data to be certain. The only reason to add it to lotion is to cut costs. It is used as a skin conditioner and humectant, and there are plenty of natural alternatives.

◇ panthenol: Some studies have shown organ effects and skin sensitivity. It depends on the form in which it is used. Some are food-grade and safe; some are not.

◇ dehydroacetic acid: This is from the material safety data sheet (MSDS) that accompanies every ingredient that you eventually purchase. It informs you about handling, employees working with it, and much more: "Hazardous in case of skin contact (irritant, sensitizer), of eye contact (irritation), of ingestion, of inhalation…may be toxic to kidneys, liver, central nervous system (CNS). Repeated or prolonged exposure…can produce target organs damage." This ingredient is considered toxic by most reliable studies and sources.

◇ benzyl alcohol: From the MSDS: "Harmful if swallowed, inhaled, or absorbed through the skin. Causes irritation to skin, eyes, and respiratory tract. Affects central nervous system." This ingredient is considered toxic by most reliable studies and informational resources.

Key to Ingredient Ratings	
S = safe	**?** = not enough data
P = potentially harmful	**H** = harmful

S	water	S: 23
S	almond (*Prunus amygdalus*) oil	P: 7
P	caprylic/capric triglyceride	H: 1
P	emulsifying wax NF	
P	sea algae extract	
S	glycerin	
S	shea (*Butyrospermum parkii*) butter	
S	avocado (*Persea americana*) oil	
P	sodium PCA	
S	aloe (*Aloe barbadensis*) gel	
S	panthenol	
S	sodium hyaluronate	
P	yeast (*Saccharomyces lysate*) extract	
P	yucca (*Yucca glauca*) extract	
S	wheat germ (*Triticum vulgare*) oil	
S	borage (*Borago officinalis*) seed oil	
S	sclerotium (*Sclerotium rolfssii*) gum powder	
S	prairie sage (*Artemisia ludoviciana*) oil	
S	sage (*Salvia officinalis*) oil	
S	Douglas fir (*Pseudotsuga menziesii*) oil	
S	lavender (*Lavandula angustifolia*) oil	
S	litsea (*Litsea cubeba*) oil	
S	pink grapefruit (*Citrus paradisi*) oil	
S	orange (*Citrus sinensis*) oil	
S	ylang-ylang (*Cananga odorata*) oil	
S	tocopherol (vitamin E)	
S	ascorbic acid (vitamin C)	
S	ascorbyl palmitate (vitamin C)	
S	xanthan gum	
P	dehydroacetic acid	
H	benzyl alcohol	

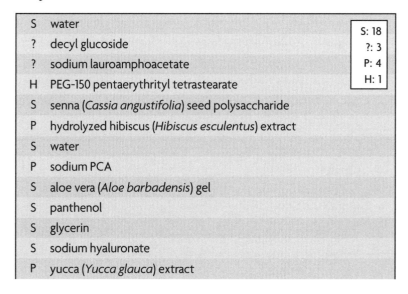

2. Encantado Shower Gel

The gel contains one known toxic ingredient (PEG-150 pentaerythrityl tetrastearate) and four questionable ones (decyl glucoside, sodium lauroamphoacetate, sodium PCA, panthenol) as well as several safe synthetics. Even though this product is safer than most on the market, I would not use it due to the presence of PEG-150.

Let's take a closer look:

◇ decyl glucoside: Considered a safe synthetic, this goes through extensive processing to become a lathering agent. There isn't enough data at this point to know whether it is truly safe.

◇ sodium lauroamphoacetate: A synthetic surfactant, this can cause some skin irritation. There hasn't been much recent research, but some studies suggest it is an organ-system carcinogen.

◇ PEG-150 (pentaerythrityl tetrastearate): Linked to organ-system toxicity and possible contamination from ethylene oxide and 1,4-dioxane. Definitely toxic and not natural, this is a chemical that is on my "avoid" list.

◇ sodium PCA: See above.

◇ panthenol: See above.

S	water	S: 18
?	decyl glucoside	?: 3
?	sodium lauroamphoacetate	P: 4
H	PEG-150 pentaerythrityl tetrastearate	H: 1
S	senna (*Cassia angustifolia*) seed polysaccharide	
P	hydrolyzed hibiscus (*Hibiscus esculentus*) extract	
S	water	
P	sodium PCA	
S	aloe vera (*Aloe barbadensis*) gel	
S	panthenol	
S	glycerin	
S	sodium hyaluronate	
P	yucca (*Yucca glauca*) extract	

S	prairie sage (*Artemisia ludoviciana*) oil
S	lavender (*Lavandula angustifolia*) oil
S	Douglas fir (*Pseudotsuga menziesii*) oil
S	petitgrain (*Citrus aurantium*) oil
S	pink grapefruit (*Citrus paradisi*) oil
S	black spruce (*Picea mariana*) oil
S	sage (*Salvia officinalis*) oil
S	ylang-ylang (*Cananga odorata*) oil
S	spearmint (*Mentha spicata*) oil
S	litsea (*Litsea cubeba*) oil
S	citric acid
?	gluconolactone
P	sodium benzoate

3. Tom's of Maine Orange-Mango Toothpaste

◇ sodium fluoride: Too much controversy to list; I'm neutral. (See Chapter 9 for a discussion on sodium fluoride.)

◇ sodium lauryl sulfate: Studies suggest it causes skin irritation and inflammation, hormone imbalance, eye irritation/eye deformities in children, and protein denaturing; it is a potential carcinogen. Additional studies suggest further health risks: SLS may mimic estrogens, cause hair loss, and damage teeth. One of the worst sources of absorption is from toothpaste and mouthwash, via the mucus membrane in the mouth. SLS can be stored in the liver, heart, lungs, and brain.

P	sodium fluoride	S:3
P	sorbitol	P: 7
P	hydrated silica	
S	water	
P	fruit extracts—mango, orange, and lemon, with other natural flavors	
P	xylitol	
P	sodium lauryl sulfate	
P	zinc citrate trihydrate	

S	xanthan gum
S	menthol

4. Encantado Shampoo and Conditioner

Although this shampoo is better than most on the market, it still contains a few harmful and questionable ingredients (such as PEG-150) that would cause me to stop using it.

Encantado Shampoo

S	water	**S: 13**
?	sodium lauroamphoacetate	**?: 4**
P	lauramidopropyl betaine	**P: 8**
?	decyl glucoside	**H: 1**
S	senna (*Cassia angustifolia*) seed polysaccharide	
P	hydrolyzed hibiscus (*Hibiscus esculentus*) extract	
?	behenamidopropyl hydroxyethyl dimonium chloride	
S	panthenol	
P	panthenol hydroxypropyl steardimonium chloride	
S	hydrolyzed rice protein	
P	burdock (*Arctium lappa*) extract	
P	ivy (*Hedera helix*) extract	
P	fenugreek (*Trigonella foenum-graecum*) extract	
P	yucca (*Yucca glauca*) extract	
H	PEG-150 pentaerythrityl tetrastearate	
S	Douglas fir (*Pseudotsuga menziesii*) oil	
S	petitgrain (*Citrus aurantium*) oil	
S	pink grapefruit (*Citrus paradisi*) oil	
S	black spruce (*Picea mariana*) oil	
S	sage (*Salvia officinalis*) oil	
S	ylang-ylang (*Cananga odorata*) oil	
S	spearmint (*Mentha spicata*) oil	
S	litsea (*Litsea cubeba*) oil	
S	citric acid	
?	gluconolactone	
P	sodium benzoate	

Encantado Conditioner

The conditioner is better than the shampoo because although it contains several potentially harmful ingredients, only the last one listed, benzyl alcohol, is harmful, making it far better than most conditioners available.

S	water	**S: 22**
P	behentrimonium methosulfate	**P: 4**
S	cetearyl alcohol	**H: 1**
S	hydrolyzed wheat protein	
S	wheat oligosaccharides	
S	panthenol	
S	linoleic acid	
S	linolenic acid	
S	hyaluronic acid	
S	sorbitol	
S	wheat germ (*Triticum vulgare*) oil	
S	jojoba (*Simmondsia chinensis*) seed oil	
S	tocopherol (vitamin E)	
P	hydrolyzed hibiscus (*Hibiscus esculentus*) extract	
P	yucca (*Yucca glauca*) extract	
S	water	
S	senna (*Cassia angustifolia*) seed polysaccharide	
S	prairie sage (*Artemisia ludoviciana*) oil	
S	sage (*Salvia officinalis*) oil	
S	Douglas fir (*Pseudotsuga menziesii*) oil	
S	lavender (*Lavandula angustifolia*) oil	
S	litsea (*Litsea cubeba*) oil	
S	pink grapefruit (*Citrus paradisi*) oil	
S	orange (*Citrus sinensis*) oil	
S	ylang-ylang (*Cananga odorata*) oil	
P	dehydroacetic acid	
H	benzyl alcohol	

5. Sumbody Lucky Lips Unscented Lip Balm

Completely pure and safe.

S	shea (*Butyrospermum parkii*) butter	**S: 7**
S	apricot (*Prunus armeniaca*) oil	
S	pistachio (*Pistacia vera*) oil	
S	beeswax (*Cera alba*)	
S	castor (*Ricinus communis*) bean oil	
S	avocado (*Persea americana*) oil	
S	jojoba (*Simmondsia chinensis*) seed oil	

6. Kerstin Florian Aromatherapy Neroli Water

It was hard to find information on this spray. I believe that the only ingredient is bitter orange flower water. If so, it is completely natural and safe.

S	bitter orange (*Citrus aurantium*) flower water	S: 1

7. Sumbody Get Lei'd Pure Sense Roll-On Perfume

Listing an ingredient as "Sumscent blend" can theoretically be done to obscure the actual ingredients. I don't like this type of labeling because it makes it easy for the manufacturer to hide fragrances in what they call the blend (the term "scent blend" does not give you enough information for you to know if there is fragrance in the product or not). Because of this, we are changing all our labels so the consumer will know if any of our blends contain synthetic fragrance. This particular scent blend does contain a very small amount of fragrance—less than 10 percent, which is much less than most scents with synthetic fragrance. Fragrances are hard for people to give up because they get attached to a scent and cannot switch. I recommend trying a pure essential-oil blend, and if you just can't find one you like, Get Lei'd is a perfect compromise, since the essential oils contained in it are suspended in pure jojoba oil and the product only has a small amount of fragrance.

S	jojoba (*Simmondsia chinensis*) seed oil	S: 1
P	Sumbody's Sumscent Blend	P: 1

8. Arcona Triad Pads (face-cleaning pads)

This product looks good and clean. The only thing to question is what the extracts it contains are extracted in.

I called the company to find out, but the company representative refused to give a clear answer as to what substance these ingredients are extracted in.

S	witch hazel (*Hamamelis virginiana*) extract	S: 5
S	rice milk	P: 4
P	sodium lactate	
P	cranberry (*Vaccinium macrocarpon*) extract	
P	white tea (*Camellia sinensis*) extract	
P	grape (*Vitis vinifera*) seed extract	
S	alpha-tocopherol (vitamin E)	
S	citric acid	
S	essential oils	

9. Tom's of Maine Original Unscented Deodorant

Unfortunately, this deodorant contains many harmful ingredients. While many people believe the brand is pure and natural, it is just as toxic as most other deodorants on the market. It contains propylene glycol, which is on my "Top Ten Ingredients to Avoid" list (see page 32).

◇ propylene glycol: A cosmetic form of mineral oil found in automatic brakes, hydraulic fluid, and industrial antifreeze. In the skin and hair, propylene glycol works as a humectant, which prevents the escape of moisture or water. The MSDS warns users to avoid skin contact with propylene glycol, as it can cause liver abnormalities and kidney damage, as well as eye irritation, skin irritation, skin drying, and defatting. Ingestion causes similar complications. Although exposure to high levels of propylene glycol is known to cause serious and potentially irreversible health conditions, the chemical industry tells us that "small" quantities or low-level exposure is "safe" on the skin and in food. According to the safety data sheets of industrial-chemical manufacturers, chemicals such as ethylene glycol and propylene glycol will cause serious health conditions, including heart damage and damage to the central nervous system if a sufficient amount is absorbed by the body. They act as a surfactant (wetting agent and solvent). They easily penetrate the skin and can weaken protein and cellular structure and are commonly used to make extracts from herbs. Propylene glycol is strong enough to remove barnacles from boats! The Environmental Protection Agency considers it so toxic that it requires workers to wear protective gloves, clothing, and goggles and to dispose of any PG solutions by burying them in the ground. But there isn't even a warning label on products such as deodorant sticks, where the concentration is greater than in most industrial applications.

H	propylene glycol	S: 6
S	water	P: 3
P	sodium stearate	H: 1
S	organic aloe vera (*Aloe barbadensis*) leaf juice	
S	witch hazel (*Hamamelis virginiana*) water	
P	glyceryl laurate	
S	chamomile aqueous extract	
P	hops (*Humulus lupulus*) extract	
S	ascorbic acid (vitamin C)	
S	organic lemongrass oil (*Cymbopogon* sp.)	

10. CleanWell All-Natural Hand Wash

Contains propylene glycol (see #9, above) and "-cones" (see #12, below), as well as other harmful ingredients.

S	ethyl alcohol	S: 4
S	water	?: 2
P	stearyl alcohol	P: 9
P	cyclomethicone	H: 4
P	C12-15 alkyl benzoate	
?	cetyl lactate	
P	cocamidopropyl PG-dimonium chloride phosphate	
S	glycerin	
H	PEG-4	

H	propylene glycol
S	tocopherol (vitamin E) acetate
?	aminomethyl propanol
P	carbomer
P	styrene/acrylates copolymer
H	fragrance
H	diazolidinyl urea
P	iodopropynyl butylcarbamate
P	methylparaben
P	propylparaben

11. CleanWell All-Natural Hand Sanitizer

S	thyme (*Thymus vulgaris*) oil	S: 8
S	aloe (*Aloe barbadensis*) leaf juice	P: 2
S	citric acid	H: 1
S	orange (*Citrus sinensis*) oil	
H	copper PCA	
P	dicapryl sodium sulfosuccinate	
S	hydrolyzed oats (*Avena sativa*)	
S	litsea (*Litsea cubeba*) oil	
S	oregano (*Origanum vulgare*) oil	
P	sodium citrate	
S	water	

12. MD Skincare Hydra-Pure Firming Eye Cream

This is filled with not only harmful ingredients but also ones known to accelerate the aging process. The "-cones" feel absolutely wonderful on your skin, which is why they are so widely used, but they cause damage in the long run. Avoid them at all costs.

- dimethicone
- dimethicone copolyol
- cyclomethicone
- silicone
- sodium PCA (see #1, above)

Let's take a closer look at a few -cones.

◇ cyclomethicone: Silicone emollients such as cyclomethicone are occlusive—that is, they coat the skin, trapping anything beneath it, and prevent it from breathing (much like plastic wrap would do). They also trap rancid oils, dirt, and grime, causing collagen to deteriorate and speeding up the aging process, leaving skin looking older than it is. Recent studies have indicated that prolonged exposure of the skin to sweat, by occlusion, causes skin irritation. Some synthetic emollients are known tumor promoters and accumulate in the liver and lymph nodes. They are also nonbiodegradable, causing negative environmental impact.

◇ silicone: Used as breast implants. Tens of thousands of women with breast implants have complained of debilitating symptoms. Anecdotal evidence indicates silicone to be toxic to the human body.

◇ sodium PCA: Linked to cancer and may be contaminated with other toxic impurities.

S	purified water	S: 15
P	cyclomethicone	?: 1
S	glycerin	P: 4
P	sodium PCA	
P	gamma-aminobutyric acid	
?	palmitoyl tetrapeptide-7	
S	sodium hyaluronate	
S	ascorbyl palmitate (vitamin C)	
S	retinol	
S	retinol (vitamin A) palmitate	
S	tocopherol (vitamin E) acetate	
S	ubiquinone	
P	emblic (*Phyllanthus emblica*) extract	
S	genistein (soy isoflavones)	
S	lycopene	
S	evening primrose (*Oenothera biennis*) essential oil	
S	olive (*Olea europaea*) oil	

S	sweet almond (*Prunus amygdalus dulcis*) oil
S	lavender (*Lavandula angustifolia*) essential oil
S	squalene

13. Skin Authority Vitamin A Cell Renewal

Overall, I found this brand to be the worst offender in Tracy's daily routine, not only because of the level of toxins but also because of the damage to skin. This product boasts the antiaging and antiacne properties of vitamin A. Unfortunately, the chemicals it contains undo any benefits the vitamin A could possibly confer. These ingredients contain chemicals such as ethylhexyl methoxycinnamate and phenoxyethanol. Ethylhexyl methoxycinnamate is known to be toxic, and even the chemical lobbyists do not dispute this. They do, however, argue that even though it is proven to be toxic, it cannot penetrate skin and therefore will not harm you. Phenoxyethanol (from the MSDS sheet) is harmful if swallowed, inhaled, or absorbed through the skin. It may cause reproductive defects, and it is a severe eye and skin irritant. Some other names it goes by are arosol, dowanol EP, dowanol EPH, emery 6705, ethylene glycol phenyl ether, ethylene glycol monophenyl ether, phenoxetol, phenoxyethanol, phenoxyethyl alcohol, 1-hydroxy-2-phenoxyethane, 2-phenoxyethanol, glycol monophenyl ether, phenylmonoglycol ether, rose ether, and beta-hydroxyethyl phenyl ether. It is important to know all the synonyms of chemicals you want to avoid, since, as you can see, a chemical can be listed in many ways. The stance I have taken in this book by rating this ingredient as harmful and parabens as potentially harmful may confuse some readers. It is important to get the message across that one should not eliminate one bad chemical and replace it with another that is equally bad or potentially worse.

S	water	S: 10
S	retinol (vitamin A) palmitate	?: 2
S	sweet almond (*Prunus amygdalus dulcis*) oil	P: 15
?	dicaprylate/dicaprate	H: 5
?	C12-15 alkyl benzoate	

S	tocopherol (vitamin E) acetate
H	propylene glycol
H	ethylhexyl methoxycinnamate
S	stearic acid
P	glyceryl stearate SE
S	aloe (*Aloe barbadensis*) leaf juice
P	birch (*Betula alba*) bark extract
P	chamomile (*Matricaria recutita*) extract
P	comfrey (*Symphytum officinale*) extract
P	ivy (*Hedera helix*) extract
P	marsh mallow (*Althaea officinalis*) root extract
S	tocopherol (vitamin E)
S	corn (*Zea mays*) oil
S	hydrolyzed soy protein
S	cetyl esters
P	polysorbate-80
P	sorbitan oleate
P	carbomer
P	disodium EDTA
P	acrylamide/ammonium acrylate copolymer
P	polyisobutene
P	polysorbate-20
H	triethanolamine
H	phenoxyethanol
P	caprylyl glycol
H	hexylene glycol
P	ethylhexyl glycerin

14. Skin Authority Sunscreen Moisturizer

It is extremely hard to find a clean sunscreen. There is a lot of controversy concerning the active ingredients generally used in sunscreens, and many of the most commonly used ingredients mimic our bodies' hormones and are known or suspected carcinogens.

Active ingredients

P	avobenzone	
H	homosalate	S: 6
H	octinoxate	?: 0
H	octisalate	P: 17
H	octocrylene	H: 9
H	oxybenzone	

Other ingredients

S	water
S	starch
P	SD alcohol-40
P	C12-15 alkyl benzoate
P	dipropylene glycol dibenzoate
P	PPG-15 stearyl ether benzoate
P	butyloctyl salicylate
P	cyclomethicone
H	PEG/PPG-18/18 dimethicone
P	silica
P	VP/hexadecane copolymer
S	aloe (*Aloe barbadensis*) leaf juice
p	algae extract
S	panthenol
S	tocopherol (vitamin E) acetate
S	tocopherol (vitamin E)
P	dimethicone
P	polysorbate-80
P	isostearic acid
H	triethanolamine (TEA)
P	tetrasodium EDTA
P	acrylates/C10-30 alkyl acrylate crosspolymer
H	phenoxyethanol
P	caprylyl glycol
P	ethylhexyl glycerin
H	hexylene glycol

15. Skin Authority Resurfacing Accelerator

This is one of this brand's cleaner products, but it is still filled with harmful synthetics.

S	water	S: 2
P	glycolic acid	P: 7
P	hydroxyethyl cellulose	H: 2
P	Canadian willowherb (*Epilobium angustifolium*) extract	
P	sodium hydroxide	
S	allantoin	
P	tetrasodium EDTA	
H	phenoxyethanol	
P	caprylyl glycol	
P	ethylhexyl glycerin	
H	hexylene glycol	

16. Skin Authority Tri-Power Peptide Hydrator

S	water	S: 13
P	C12-15 alkyl benzoate	?: 3
H	dipropylene glycol dibenzoate	P: 16
H	hydroxyethyl cellulose	H: 7
S	glycerin	
P	algae extract	
?	phenyl trimethicone	
P	cyclomethicone	
?	polysilicone-11	
S	lecithin	
S	sodium hyaluronate	
P	glyceryl stearate	
H	PEG-100 stearate	
P	DEA-cetyl phosphate	
P	glyceryl stearate	
S	stearic acid	
S	cetearyl alcohol	
S	palmitoyl hydrolyzed wheat protein	

S	phytosqualene
S	panthenol
S	tocopherol (vitamin E) linoleate
S	pyridoxine (vitamin B-6)
P	tetrahexyldecyl ascorbate
S	dipalmitoyl hydroxyproline
P	stearyl glycyrrhetinate
S	tocopherol (vitamin E)
H	butylene glycol
P	carbomer
P	polysorbate-20
?	acetyl hexapeptide-8
P	palmitoyl oligopeptide
P	palmitoyl tetrapeptide-7
P	alkyl acrylate crosspolymer
H	phenoxyethanol
P	caprylyl glycol
P	ethylhexyl glycerin
H	hexylene glycol
P	ethylenediaminetetraacetic acid (EDTA)
H	triethanolamine (TEA)

17. Skin Authority Daily Cleanser

This product has eleven ingredients, nine of which are harmful or potentially harmful. The only safe ingredients are water and sodium chloride (salt).

S	water	S: 2
P	sodium laureth sulfate	?: 0
H	cocamidopropyl betaine	P: 7
H	PEG-150 pentaerythrityl tetrastearate	H: 2
P	glycolic acid	
P	disodium cocoamphodiacetate	
P	hydroxyethyl cellulose	
P	disodium EDTA	

P	methylchloroisothiazolinone
P	methylisothiazolinone
S	sodium chloride

18. Skin Authority AOX C&E Lip Therapy

I would avoid this product because not only is it absorbed through your skin, but since it is applied to your lips, you ingest some of it as well. It contains a paraben preservative and mineral oil, which is petroleum-based and tends to create an addictive need—if you do not apply it, your lips will become dry and chapped. It also contains bismuth oxychloride, which is counterproductive for skin (i.e., it reverses the benefits created by the other good ingredients in the product).

Active ingredients

S	L-ascorbic acid	S: 6	
S	vitamin E	P: 3	

Inactive ingredients

S	castor (*Ricinus communis*) bean oil
S	beeswax (*Cera alba*)
P	mineral oil
S	carnauba (*Copernicia cerifera*) wax
S	candelilla (*Euphorbia antisyphilitica*) wax
P	bismuth oxychloride
P	paraben

19. California Baby Calming Aromatherapy Bubble Bath

I know bubble bath is fun, but unfortunately I would suggest other fun things for a baby's bath. Not only is there no good alternative bubble bath, but bubble baths are designed for soaking, which lengthens exposure to harmful chemicals. While this brand is better than most, I would discontinue or severely limit my use of it.

Also, most of the California Baby products contain the following ingredient:

◈ Proprietary Broad Spectrum Protection Preservative System. We have no way of knowing what this means. I contacted them several times and spoke to different people, and the company refused to explain it to me.

S	purified water		S: 11
P	decyl polyglucose		?: 1
S	soapbark (*Quillaja saponaria*)		P: 1
S	yucca (*Yucca glauca*)		
S	calendula (*Calendula officinalis*)		
S	aloe vera (*Aloe barbadensis*)		
S	rose (*Rosa canina*) water		
S	cactus		
S	acacia (*Acacia* sp.)		
S	Irish moss (*Chondrus crispus*)		
S	vitamin E		
S	proprietary calming essential oil blend		
?	proprietary broad-spectrum protection preservative system		

Note: California Baby lists ingredients such as Irish moss and yucca without saying that they are in an extract; I am giving them the benefit of the doubt that they are correctly listed and calling it safe. The only other option besides an extract for some of the ingredients they have listed is to make a tea in the water and strain it. Since Irish moss and yucca are not dissolvable, adding the herb in a powder form, unless in minute amounts, would not work.

20. California Baby Calming Everyday Lotion

This product contains methylparaben, which mimics estrogen and has been found in breast cancer tumors, as well as some other questionable ingredients. There are wonderful lotions that are all natural; you don't need to use products labeled specifically for babies on your infant. Pure butters are also soft and nourishing for baby skin.

S	purified water		S: 15
P	caprylic/capric triglyceride		?: 2
S	apricot (*Prunus armeniaca*) oil		P: 2

S	aloe vera (*Aloe barbadensis*)
S	yucca (*Yucca glauca*)
S	rose (*Rosa canina*) water
S	rose hips (*Rosa canina*)
S	cactus
S	chamomile (*Matricaria recutita*)
S	acacia (*Acacia* sp.)
S	Irish moss (*Chondrus crispus*)
S	vitamin E
S	proprietary calming essential oil blend
?	proprietary broad-spectrum protection preservative system that includes antibacterial essential oils
S	vitamin A
S	vitamin C
S	vitamin E
?	small amount of food-grade preservatives
P	methylparaben

21. California Baby Calming Shampoo & Bodywash

This product contains:

◇ decyl polyglucose (extracts of corn, coconut, palm). As mentioned previously, there is nothing perfect in this category, so if you love this product, stick with it. It is better than most. I would also wash babies' hair only when it really needs it, limiting exposure.

S	water (purified)	S: 6
S	aloe vera (*Aloe barbadensis*)	P: 2
P	decyl polyglucose (extracts of corn, coconut, palm)	
S	vitamin E	
S	vegetable glycerin	
S	jojoba (*Simmondsia chinensis*) seed oil	
P	citrus seed extract	
S	vitamin B-5	

22. California Baby SPF 30+ Sunblock Stick

This sunblock contains:

◇ ozokerite: Irritant to eyes, skin, and lungs, in addition to being linked to organ system toxicity.

◇ propylparaben: Propylparaben is inked to developmental and reproductive toxicity, endocrine disruption, immunotoxicity, and organ system toxicity. It also aggravates allergies, sensitizes skin, and poses an environmental hazard.

While this brand is better than the Nature's Gate (see #23 below), I will later suggest a cleaner one.

P	micronized titanium dioxide	S: 4
P	caprylic/capric triglyceride	P: 4
S	candelilla (*Euphorbia antisyphilitica*) wax	
S	carnauba (*Copernica cerifera*) wax	
S	beeswax (*Cera alba*)	
P	ozokerite	
S	vitamin E	
P	propylparaben	

23. Nature's Gate Kid's Block 30 SPF Sunscreen

I would suggest not using this product, as it contains many harmful ingredients (see below).

Active ingredients

H	octinoxate	S: 5
H	octocrylene	?: 3
H	oxybenzone	P: 8
S	titanium dioxide	H: 7

Inactive ingredients

S	water
S	certified organic lavender (*Lavender angustifolia*) flower/leaf/stem extract
?	solarium complex (phatania, coffee, and wild pansy extracts; pycnogenol; extracts of kola nut, aloe barbadensis, suma, strawflower, alder buckthorn, and chamomile)

P	sorbitol
P	VP/eicosene copolymer
P	ethylhexyl palmitate
P	PEG-100 Stearate
?	bisabolol
S	cetearyl alcohol
H	ceteareth-20
P	glyceryl undecylenate
?	ethylhexyl glycerin
S	glycerin
H	triethanolamine
P	tromethamine
P	carbomer
P	dimethicone
H	fragrance
H	phenoxyethanol

24. Erbaviva Diaper Cream

This product contains:

◇ sodium hydroxymethylglycinate: In aqueous solution, this decomposes to sodium glycinate and formaldehyde. From the MSDS: "Skin Contact: Immediately wash with soap and plenty of water. Remove contaminated clothing and launder before reuse. Get medical attention if symptoms occur."

S	deionized water	S: 10
P	zinc oxide	P: 4
S	organic almond (*Prunus amygdalus*) oil	
S	avocado (*Persea americana*) oil	
S	cetearyl wheat bran glycosides	
S	cetearyl alcohol	
P	echinacea (*Echinacea purpurea*) extract	
S	lecithin	
P	algae extract	
S	beeswax (*Cera alba*)	

S	allantoin
P	sodium hydroxymethylglycinate
S	organic lavender (*Lavandula angustifolia*) essential oil
S	organic Roman chamomile (*Anthemis nobilis*) essential oil

25. California Baby Diaper Area Wash

S	purified water	**S: 6**
S	witch hazel (*aqua hamamelis/Hamamelis virginiana*)	
S	calendula (*Calendula officinalis*)	
S	aloe vera (*Aloe barbadensis*)	
S	tea tree (organic) (*Melaleuca alternifolia*)	
S	essential oil blend	

If I have listed an ingredient as harmful, there is an overwhelming amount of data that verifies the ingredient is toxic. These are not controversial assumptions. This evaluation will be considered very conservative by most experts concerned with the harmful effects of toxic chemicals in personal-care products; they would also put all of my "potentially harmful" ingredients in the "harmful" list. If I've labeled an ingredient "potentially harmful," there are data and studies that indicate that the chemical is harmful, but not enough research has been done to make a conclusive statement. When it comes to potential toxic exposure, I promote a guilty-until-proven-innocent policy and advocate that chemical manufacturers do the research and prove an ingredient is safe before it goes on the market. As it stands now, anything goes and it is extremely difficult to get ingredients taken off the market in the cosmetic industry.

Additionally, there has been no research on the effect of all these chemicals mixing in your bloodstream. We also do not know about effects over time, and whether or not the toxins stored in fat cells can build up to a harmful level.

I try to focus on moderation and solutions. With that said, if there are some products in your daily routine that you just cannot give up, keep them. Our goal is to lower your overall exposure. Any changes you make will have a positive effect. Any product you soak in, leave on for considerable lengths of time, or put on your lips would be my first to go.

Here are some additional things to keep in mind when looking at labels and searching for products:

◇ Extracts that don't specify what the herb is extracted with are suspect. This is a way that companies can hide ingredients. For this reason I listed them as potential.

◇ Certain types of alcohol I have listed as potentially harmful. When it came to listing these, I vacillated between "safe" and "potentially harmful," since there is a lot of controversy in the research. On one hand, alcohol in large quantities is not good for you or your skin; on the other hand, it is great in small quantities for its antibacterial and preservative properties, and for its use in the extraction of herbs.

◇ Note on essential oils: I have them listed as most studies list them. They are, however, one of the natural ingredients with the highest amount of allergic reaction. Also you will see ingredients on labels such as limonene, linalool, coumarin, and cintronellal. If you research them, you will find them listed as harmful in some studies. I listed them as safe. They are naturally occurring components of the essential oil. Use all essential oils with caution, keep away from mucus glands, and test a small area of your skin with the product before using.

Current Product Profile
Tracy

◇ 18 products

◇ 319 total ingredients (some redundant, i.e., same ingredient in different products)

◇ 159 safe (S)   ◇ 13 not enough data (?)

◇ 113 potentially harmful (P)   ◇ 34 harmful (H)

Baby

- ◇ 7 products
- ◇ 65 safe (S)
- ◇ 21 potentially harmful (P)
- ◇ 101 total ingredients
- ◇ 7 not enough data (?)
- ◇ 8 harmful (H)

That was the complete ingredient profile of the products Tracy was using before her makeover. The following are the healthful alternatives to which she switched.

Replacement Product Profile (product descriptions to follow)

- ◇ 16 products
- ◇ 288 safe (S)
- ◇ 9 potentially harmful (P)
- ◇ 305 total ingredients
- ◇ 8 not enough data (?)
- ◇ 0 harmful (H)

Key to Ingredient Ratings	
S = safe	**?** = not enough data
P = potentially harmful	**H** = harmful

1. Sumbody Be Fresh Body Deodorant (replaces Tom's of Maine Original Unscented Deodorant)

S	distilled water	S: 5
S	witch hazel (*Hamamelis virginiana*) distillate	P: 1
S	aloe vera (*Aloe barbadensis*) juice	
P	organic grape (*Vitis labrusca*) alcohol	
S	mineral salts	
S	Sum Essential Oil Blend	

2. Sumbody Pure Sense Roll-On Perfume: Citrus Splash, Lavender, Ice Queen, Sweet and Sassy, Wild Thing, Daredevil (replaces Sumbody Get Lei'd Pure Sense Roll-On Perfume)

S	jojoba (*Simmondsia chinensis*) seed oil	S: 2
S	Sum Essential Oil Blend	

3. Sumbody A–Z Face Cream (replaces Skin Authority Vitamin A Cell Renewal and Skin Authority Sunscreen Moisturizer)

S	water	S: 31
P	emulsifying wax	?: 1
S	stearic acid	P: 3

S   olive (*Olea europaea*) oil

S   organic aloe (*Aloe barbadensis*) leaf juice

S   vitamin A

S   vitamin C ester

S   wolfberry (*Lycium barbarum*) extract, extracted in jojoba oil

S   shiitake mushroom (*Lentinus edodes*) extract, extracted in jojoba oil

S   bamboo (*Bambusa* sp.) extract, extracted in jojoba oil

S   pomegranate (*Punica granatum*) extract, extracted in jojoba oil

S   rooibos (*Aspalathus linearis*) extract, extracted in jojoba oil

S   hibiscus (*Hibiscus sabdariffa*) extract, extracted in jojoba oil

S   asafetida (*Ferula foetida*) extract, extracted in jojoba oil

S   pear (*Pyrus communis*) extract, extracted in jojoba oil

S   white tea (*Camellia sinensis*) extract, extracted in jojoba oil

S   black tea (*Camellia sinensis*) extract, extracted in jojoba oil

S   green tea (*Camellia sinensis*) extract, extracted in jojoba oil

S   Himalayan raspberry (*Rubus ellipticus*) root extract, extracted in jojoba oil

S   hazelnut (*Corylus avellana*) extract, extracted in jojoba oil

S   thale cress (*Arabidopsis thaliana*) extract, extracted in jojoba oil

S   seaweed (*Fucus vesiculosis*)

S   lecithin

S   carrot (*Daucus carota sativa*) seed oil

P   alpha-lipoic acid

S   methylsulfonylmethane (MSM)

S   wheat (*Triticum vulgare*) amino acids

S   oat (*Avena sativa*) amino acids

S   vitamin E

P   zinc oxide

S	neem (*Melia azadirachta*) seed oil
S	rosemary (*Rosmarinus officinalis*) oil
S	black willow (*Salix nigra*) bark extract, extracted in jojoba oil
S	lichen (*Usnea barbata*) extract, extracted in jojoba oil
?	potassium sorbate

4. Sumbody Mineral Foundation (replaces the Skin Authority Sunscreen Moisturizer)

S	mica	S: 30
S	boron nitride	
S	titanium dioxide	
S	silica microspheres	
S	magnesium stearate	
S	pearl powder	
S	silk powder	
S	shea (*Butyrospermum parkii*) butter	
S	calendula (*Calendula officinalis*) extract, extracted in jojoba oil	
S	lavender (*Lavandula angustifolia*) extract, extracted in jojoba oil	
S	green tea (*Camellia sinensis*) extract, extracted in jojoba oil	
S	white tea (*Camellia sinensis*) extract, extracted in jojoba oil	
S	rooibos (*Aspalathus linearis*) extract, extracted in jojoba oil	
S	chamomile (*Matricaria recutita*) extract, extracted in jojoba oil	
S	licorice (*Glykyrrhiza glabra*) root extract, extracted in jojoba oil	
S	horsetail (*Equisetum arvense*) extract, extracted in jojoba oil	
S	chestnut (*Castanea sativa*) extract, extracted in jojoba oil	
S	chrysanthemum (*Chrysanthemum* sp.) extract, extracted in jojoba oil	
S	burdock (*Arctium lappa*) extract, extracted in jojoba oil	
S	nettle (*Urtica dioica*) extract, extracted in jojoba oil	
S	rose (*Rosa canina*) extract extracted in jojoba oil	
S	orrisroot (*Iris germanica*) extract, extracted in jojoba oil	
S	spirulina (*Arthrospira platensis*) extract, extracted in jojoba oil	
S	bladder wrack (*Fucus vesiculosus*) extract, extracted in jojoba oil	
S	kombu (*Laminaria japonica*) extract, extracted in jojoba oil	

S	shiitake mushroom (*Lentinus edodes*) extract, extracted in jojoba oil
S	Irish moss (*Chondrus crispus*) extract, extracted in jojoba oil
S	juniper (*Juniperus communis*) berry extract, extracted in jojoba oil
S	kelp (*Ascophyllum nodosum*) extract, extracted in jojoba oil
S	carrot (*Daucus carota sativa*) seed oil

5. Sumbody Skin Tight Face Serum (replaces Skin Authority Resurfacing Accelerator and MD Skincare Hydra-Pure Firming Eye Cream)

S	chamomile (*Matricaria recutita*) flower water	S: 35
P	emulsifying wax	?: 1
S	coconut (*Cocos nucifera*) oil	P: 1
S	sweet almond (*Prunus amygdalus dulcis*) oil	
S	wheat germ (*Triticum vulgare*) oil	
S	stearic acid	
S	algae extract, extracted in jojoba oil	
S	kosher vegetable glycerin	
S	biosaccharide gum-1	
S	sodium hyaluronate	
S	organic aloe (*Aloe barbadensis*) leaf juice	
S	goat milk	
S	oat (*Avena sativa*) extract, extracted in jojoba oil	
S	green tea (*Camellia sinensis*) extract, extracted in jojoba oil	
S	squalene	
S	comfrey (*Symphytum officinale*) leaf extract, extracted in jojoba oil	
S	horsetail (*Equisetum arvense*) extract, extracted in jojoba oil	
S	gingko (*Ginkgo biloba*) extract, extracted in jojoba oil	
S	licorice (*Glykyrrhiza glabra*) root extract, extracted in jojoba oil	
S	plantain (*Plantago* sp.) seed extract, extracted in jojoba oil	
S	marsh mallow (*Althaea officinalis*) extract, extracted in jojoba oil	
S	rose hip (*Rosa canina*) oil	
S	pumpkin (*Cucurbita pepo*) seed oil	
S	cumin (*Cuminum cyminum*) oil	

S	sea buckthorn (*Hippophae rhamnoides*) extract, extracted in jojoba oil
S	mullein (*Verbascum thapsus*) extract, extracted in jojoba oil
S	chickweed (*Stellaria media*) extract, extracted in jojoba oil
S	fenugreek (*Trigonella foenum-graecum*) extract, extracted in jojoba oil
S	corn (*Zea mays*) silk
S	vitamin A
S	vitamin C
S	vitamin E
S	ginger (*Zingiber officinale*) extract, extracted in jojoba oil
S	neem (*Melia azadirachta*) seed oil
S	black willow (*Salix nigra*) bark extract, extracted in jojoba oil
S	lichen (*Usnea barbata*) extract, extracted in jojoba oil
?	potassium sorbate

6. Sumbody It's About Time Face Serum (replaces Skin Authority Tri-Power Peptide Hydrator)

S	rose hydrosol	S: 24
S	meadowfoam (*Limnanthes alba*) seed oil	?: 1
?	dimethylaminoethanol (DMAE)	P: 2
S	vitamin C	
P	emulsifying wax NF	
S	aloe (*Aloe barbadensis*) juice	
S	kosher vegetable glycerin	
S	vitamin E	
P	alpha-lipoic acid	
S	coenzyme Q-10	
S	lecithin	
S	vitamin A	
S	provitamin A	
S	xanthan gum	
S	neem (*Melia azadirachta*) seed oil	
S	bilberry (*Vaccinium myrtillus*) extract, extracted in jojoba oil	

S	sugarcane (*Saccharum officinrum*) extract, extracted in jojoba oil
S	sugar maple (*Acer saccharum*) extract, extracted in jojoba oil
S	orange (*Citrus sinensis*) extract, extracted in jojoba oil
S	lemon (*Citrus medica limonum*) extract, extracted in jojoba oil
S	cranberry (*Vaccinium macrocarpon*) oil
S	red raspberry (*Rubus* sp.) oil
S	evening primrose (*Oenothera biennis*) oil
S	rose hip (*Rosa canina*) oil
S	rosemary (*Rosmarinus officinalis*) leaf extract, extracted in jojoba oil
S	black willow (*Salix nigra*) bark extract, extracted in jojoba oil
S	lichen (*Usnea barbata*) extract, extracted in jojoba oil

7. Sumbody C Me Glow Face Cleanser: Normal/Dry (replaces Skin Authority Daily Cleanser)

S	German chamomile (*Matricaria recutita*) flower water	S: 18
S	aloe (*Aloe barbadensis*) leaf juice	P: 1
P	emulsifying wax	
S	burdock (*Arctium lappa*) extract, extracted in jojoba oil	
S	orrisroot (*Iris germanica*) extract, extracted in jojoba oil	
S	evening primrose (*Oenothera biennis*) oil	
S	rose hip (*Rosa canina*) oil	
S	bilberry (*Vaccinium myrtillus*) extract, extracted in jojoba oil	
S	sugarcane (*Saccharum officinarum*) extract, extracted in jojoba oil	
S	sugar maple (*Acer saccharum*) extract, extracted in jojoba oil	
S	orange (*Citrus sinensis*) extract, extracted in jojoba oil	
S	lemon (*Citrus medica limonum*) extract, extracted in jojoba oil	
S	rosemary (*Rosmarinus officinalis*) leaf extract, extracted in jojoba oil	
S	vitamin E	
S	xanthan gum	
S	neem (*Melia azadirachta*) seed oil	
S	black willow (*Salix nigra*) bark extract, extracted in jojoba oil	
S	lichen (*Usnea barbata*) extract, extracted in jojoba oil	
S	calendula (*Calendula officinalis*) extract, extracted in jojoba oil	

8. Eye'm in Love (replaces Skin Authority AOX C&E Lip Therapy and MD Skincare Firming Eye Cream)

S	pistachio (*Pistacia vera*) oil	S: 30
S	shea (*Butyrospermum parkii*) butter	
S	castor (*Ricinus communis*) seed oil	
S	apricot (*Prunus armeniaca*) oil	
S	avocado (*Persea americana*) oil	
S	jojoba (*Simmondsia chinensis*) seed oil	
S	beeswax (*Cera alba*)	
S	carrot (*Daucus carota sativa*) seed oil	
S	rose hip (*Rosa canina*) oil	
S	infused St. John's wort (*Hypericum perforatum*)	
S	vitamin C	
S	vitamin E	
S	calendula (*Calendula officinalis*)	
S	apple (*Malus domestica*)	
S	chamomile (*Matricaria recutita*)	
S	elder flower (*Sambucus nigra*)	
S	comfrey (*Symphytum officinale*)	
S	carrot (*Daucus carota sativa*)	
S	burdock (*Arctium lappa*)	
S	goldenseal (*Hydrastis canadensis*)	
S	Irish moss (*Chondrus crispus*), extracted in jojoba oil	
S	kombu (*Laminaria japonica*)	
S	wakame (*Undaria pinnatifida*)	
S	bladder wrack (*Fucus vesiculosus*)	
S	licorice (*Glykyrrhiza glabra*) root	
S	rose hip (*Rosa canina*)	
S	bee pollen	
S	green tea (*Camellia sinensis*)	
S	rooibos (*Aspalathus linearis*)	
S	noni (*Morinda citrifolia*)	

9. Sumbody Supernatural Body Wash (replaces Encantado Shower Gel)

S	deionized rosemary (*Rosmarinus officinalis*) water	S: 18
S	kumquat (*Citrus japonica*) extract	?: 1
S	kiwi (*Actinidia chinensis*) extract	
S	neem fruit extract (*Melia azadirachta*)	
S	chrysanthemum (*Chrysanthemum* sp.)	
?	abyssine (*Alteromonas ferment*)	
S	copaiba balsam (*Copaifera officinalis*)	
S	andiroba (*Carapa guianensis*)	
S	acai (*Euterpe oleracea*)	
S	lavender (*Lavandula angustifolia*)	
S	calendula (*Calendula officinalis*)	
S	wild oats (*Avena fatua*)	
S	honey	
S	oat (*Avena sativa*) amino acids	
S	honeysuckle (*Lonicera* sp.) flower extract, extracted in jojoba oil	
S	Japanese honeysuckle (*Lonicera japonica*) flower extract, extracted in jojoba oil	
S	hydrolyzed silk protein	
S	citric acid	
S	Sum Natural Scent Blend	

10. Head First SumShampoo: Normal/Dry (replaces Encantado Shampoo)

S	deionized rosemary (*Rosmarinus officinalis*) water	S: 19
S	kumquat (*Citrus japonica*) extract	?: 1
S	kiwi (*Actinidia chinensis*) extract	
S	neem (*Melia azadirachta*) fruit extract	
S	chrysanthemum (*Chrysanthemum* sp.)	
?	abyssine (*Alteromonas ferment*)	
S	copaiba balsam (*Copaifera officinalis*)	
S	andiroba (*Carapa guianensis*)	
S	acai (*Euterpe oleracea*)	

S	bamboo (*Bambusa* sp.)
S	lavender (*Lavandula angustifolia*)
S	calendula (*Calendula officinalis*)
S	wild oats (*Avena fatua*)
S	honey
S	oat (*Avena sativa*) amino acids
S	honeysuckle (*Lonicera* sp.) flower extract, extracted in jojoba oil
S	Japanese honeysuckle (*Lonicera japonica*) flower, extract extracted in jojoba oil
S	hydrolyzed silk protein
S	citric acid
S	Sumbody's Natural Blend

11. Head First SumConditioner: Normal/Dry (replaces Encantado Conditioner)

S	cetearyl alcohol	S: 11
P	glyceryl stearate	?: 1
S	macadamia (*Macadamia* sp.) oil	P: 1
S	cupuaçu (*Theobroma grandiflorum*) seed butter	
S	avocado (*Persea americana*) oil	
S	chrysanthemum (*Chrysanthemum* sp.)	
?	abyssine (*Alteromonas ferment*)	
S	acai (*Euterpe oleracea*)	
S	andiroba (*Carapa guianensis*)	
S	copaiba balsam (*Copaifera officinalis*)	
S	olive (*Olea europaea*) oil	
S	sweet almond (*Prunus amygdalus dulcis*) oil	
S	Sumbody's Natural Scent Blend	

12. Sumbody Goat Milk Lotion (replaces Encantado lotion and California Baby Calming Everyday Lotion)

S	water	S: 21
S	xanthan gum	?: 1

S	kosher vegetable glycerin
S	olive (*Olea europaea*) oil
S	stearic acid
S	coconut (*Cocos nucifera*) oil
S	sweet almond (*Prunus amygdalus dulcis*) oil
S	grape (*Vitis vinifera*) seed oil
S	avocado (*Persea americana*) oil
S	goat milk
S	rosemary (*Rosmarinus officinalis*) leaf extract
S	vitamin A
S	vitamin C
S	vitamin E
S	witch hazel (*Hamamelis virginiana*) distillate
S	neem (*Melia azadirachta*) seed oil
S	chrysanthemum (*Chrysanthemum* sp.)
?	abyssine (*Alteromonas ferment*)
S	copaiba balsam (*Copaifera officinalis*)
S	andiroba (*Carapa guianensis*)
S	acai (*Euterpe oleracea*)
S	potassium sorbate

13. Sumbody Supernatural Hand Wash (replaces CleanWell All-Natural Hand Sanitizer)

S	deionized rosemary (*Rosmarinus officinalis*) water	S: 18
S	kumquat (*Citrus japonica*) extract	?: 1
S	kiwi (*Actinidia chinensis*) extract	
S	neem (*Melia azadirachta*) fruit extract	
S	chrysanthemum (*Chrysanthemum* sp.)	
?	abyssine (*Alteromonas ferment*)	
S	copaiba balsam (*Copaifera officinalis*)	
S	andiroba (*Carapa guianensis*)	
S	acai (*Euterpe oleracea*)	
S	lavender (*Lavandula angustifolia*)	

S   calendula (*Calendula officinalis*)

S   wild oats (*Avena fatua*)

S   honey

S   oat (*Avena sativa*) amino acids

S   honeysuckle (*Lonicera* sp.) flower extract, extracted in jojoba oil

S   Japanese honeysuckle (*Lonicera japonica*) flower, extract extracted in jojoba oil

S   hydrolyzed silk protein

S   citric acid

S   Sumbody's Natural Scent Blend

14. Sumbody Bottoms Up Baby Butt Salve (replaces Erbaviva Diaper Cream)

S   shea (*Butyrospermum parkii*) butter   S: 17

S   castor (*Ricinus communis*) oil

S   jojoba (*Simmondsia chinensis*) seed oil

S   apricot (*Prunus armeniaca*) oil

S   pistachio (*Pistacia vera*) oil

S   almond (*Prunus amygdalus*) oil

S   beeswax (*Cera alba*)

S   avocado (*Persea americana*) oil

S   calendula (*Calendula officinalis*)

S   chamomile (*Matricaria recutita*)

S   comfrey (*Symphytum officinale*)

S   burdock (*Arctium lappa*)

S   red clover (*Trifolium pratense*)

S   plantain (*Plantago* sp.)

S   carrot (*Daucus carota sativa*)

S   avocado (*Persea americana*)

S   Sumbody's Essential Oil Blend

15. Sumbody Tiny Hiny (replaces California Baby Diaper Area Wash)

S	chamomile (*Matricaria recutita*)	S: 4
S	lavender (*Lavandula angustifolia*)	
S	witch hazel (*Hamamelis virginiana*)	
S	tea tree (*Melaleuca alternifolia*) hydrosol	

16. Sumbody Baby Be Moist Petroleum-Free Oil (another option to replace California Baby Calming Everyday Lotion)

S	pistachio (*Pistacia vera*) oil	S: 4
S	jojoba (*Simmondsia chinensis*) seed oil	
S	almond (*Prunus amygdalus*) oil	
S	Sumbody's Essential Oil Blend	

This was Tracy's response to my feedback:

Wow! I received the beautiful box of products and the amazing report about all the what-I-thought-were somewhat "natural" products. It's kind of depressing actually, but I feel better since I have some great substitute products now. Little Judi has had a little diaper rash for a few days and I started using the diaper wash that you sent. Rash disappeared almost immediately after I started using it. Thanks for everything! Can't wait to dig into that report.

The Verdict

When I first spoke with Tracy about her expectations for body products, she (along with every woman on the planet) wanted to eradicate all of her wrinkles and signs of aging. Natural or chemical, there is no product that can reverse all the effects of aging. However, there are ways to combat and retard them. This desire to suddenly look twenty years younger creates an immense amount of false hope and disappointment with the beauty industry. Tracy and I discussed the need for realistic goals and expectations. Of course, she was well aware beforehand what these were—we all just like to hold out for the possibility of eternal youth and wish there were such a solution.

When Tracy made the switch to truly natural products, she did notice a substantial luster and glow to her skin, and an evenness of tone. The switch also smoothed out some of her fine lines by restoring some of her skin's natural elasticity and firmness. Tracy maintains a healthy lifestyle that contributes to her overall health and that of her skin. She practices Bikram yoga, in which you sweat constantly, helping keep her pores clean and toxins expelled.

Over the course of her makeover, Tracy switched to 100 percent natural products. One of the first products to go was her Tom's deodorant, which she hadn't been happy with anyway; it was an easy switch. She loves the smell and results of the Sumbody deodorant. The next step was to decrease the number of creams she was using. In doing so, we not only decreased the amount of money she was spending on face and body creams but also improved her results. She noticed her skin becoming softer, smoother, and easier to moisturize. The switch also dispelled the myth that face creams that cost over two hundred dollars per ounce are more effective and contain better ingredients. Efficacy is related to the quality of ingredients—not to the price point.

Aside from benefiting her own skin, Tracy's chemical-free makeover has had a positive effect on the health of her baby's skin as well. When Tracy eliminated chemicals from her baby products, the diaper rash immediately disappeared. Her baby's skin was healthier and saved from the harmful effects of toxic chemicals. She is using many fewer products, and the makeover reminded her that babies really do not need that many products.

Tracy did her switch cold turkey and never looked back. Seeing the information on the products she was using was enough for her. She knows more than most people about natural versus chemical and was surprised how "loaded" her regime was. She wants to protect her family from chemical exposure, and she loves the results. Tracy also noticed an improvement in her overall energy level, and with no other changes in her life she feels sure it was due to her makeover. One less baby being exposed to potentially harmful chemicals, one baby's skin more moisturized, diaper rash gone, and one more happy mom with brighter, healthier, younger-looking skin. Mission accomplished!

The Mother

When I chose the women for the chemical-free makeover, I wanted to be sure to represent the widest spectrum possible in terms of career, family, and financial situation. I already had Tracy, the successful businesswoman with a baby, so for the second woman I chose Barbara, a working single mother of three operating on a budget. She was not raised with any awareness or concern about chemicals in cosmetics and body products, and although she was trying to limit her exposure, she was still fairly low on the learning curve. She represents a larger percentage of the population than Tracy does, especially of those who are searching for natural alternatives.

Barbara told me that she had never had "nice" skin. She suffered from breakouts, bumps, scars, discoloration, and dryness. Her skin is also very sensitive skin, so I knew that any product that works for her should be safe for all skin types. Additionally, her eleven-year-old daughter was beginning to have mild skin problems, so Barbara was trying to solve those as well. When I approached Barbara for this project, she was already trying to make choices to minimize her exposure to chemicals. For instance, she used the children's products her daughter used, both because she figured they would contain fewer chemicals and be gentler on her skin, and because she didn't have to spend the money to buy two types of shampoo, conditioner, and face cream. When I analyzed the products she was using, I found that she used some regular drugstore products and some higher-end products that were straining her budget. My goal was to lessen her exposure to chemicals, improve her and her daughter's skin, help her understand how to choose products on her own, and save her money.

Since Barbara was new to understanding what "natural" really means, education was key to her success. When explaining to Barbara about the ingredients she was exposing herself and her family to I wanted her to understand my frustration in rating the chemicals in her products and teach her how to assess them herself. This is something I cannot stress enough. You must not take my word; you need to find your own comfort zone. This is especially important since I feel most of what I rated as P is harmful, and I would not personally use a product with those types of P chemicals in it—there is enough evidence against them for me. You will notice that parabens, a chemical the public is shunning, are rated as a P. I would not use them, and the evidence against them is growing. There are still no conclusive answers—only controversy—and some of the chemicals that companies are now using to replace parabens are just as bad, or worse.

Some of the ingredients I have rated P I feel are safe, but if you inhale them in powder form, they can be harmful. So for Barbara's makeover I rated some ingredients S/P so she could learn to identify and understand these ingredients. Most of these ingredients are not powders when they come to you in a product, such as titanium dioxide in soap. However, when titanium dioxide is used in mineral makeup, it is still a powder. I feel the small amount you will breathe in is safer then the alternative chemical foundations available.

These are issues Barbara had to grapple with, as do most people when they decide to have a makeover. Once you open the door to this type of thinking and start to talk about it, everyone will have an opinion. Some people will tell you anything is potentially harmful, which is true when taken to the extreme, while others will only use soap and water. These are issues that only you can decide for yourself.

Current Product Ingredients

- 26 products
- 141 safe (S)
- 269 potentially harmful (P)
- 525 total ingredients
- 53 not enough data (?)
- 71 harmful (H)

1. Dermalogica Multivitamin Power Firm Face Cream

P	cyclopentasiloxane	S: 5
?	BIS diglyceryl polyacyladipate-2	?: 1
P	dimethicone crosspolymer	S/P: 1
P	cetyl ethylhexanoate	P: 8
H	polyethylene	H: 1
S	tocopherol (vitamin E) acetate	
P	green tea (*Camellia sinensis*) leaf extract	

P	chamomile (*Chamomilla recutita*) extract
P	algae (*Corallina officinalis*) extract
S	safflower (*Carthamus tinctorius*) seed oil
S	grape (*Vitis vinifera*) seed oil
P	flavor
S	ascorbic acid (vitamin C)
P	glycyrrhetinic acid
S/P	boron nitride
S	retinol (vitamin A) palmitate

2. Dermalogica Essential Cleansing Solution

P	bitter orange (*Citrus aurantium*) flower extract	S:4
P	caprylic/capric triglyceride	?: 2
H	butylene glycol	P: 15
S	safflower (*Carthamus tinctorius*) oil	H: 7
H	PEG-8	
P	polysorbate-60	
P	cetyl alcohol	
?	sorbitan stearate	
H	ricinoleth-40	
S	beeswax (*Cera alba*)	
P	ceresin	
?	octyl hydroxystearate	
S	tocopherol (vitamin E) acetate	
S	ascorbyl palmitate	
P	hops (*Humulus lupulus*) extract	
P	rosemary (*Rosmarinus officinalis*) extract	
P	horsetail (*Equisetum arvense*) extract	
P	pine (*Pinus sylvestris*) cone extract	
P	lemon (*Citrus medica limonum*) extract	
H	diazolidinyl urea	
P	methylparaben	
P	propylparaben	

H	propylene glycol
P	dimethicone
H	triethanolamine (TEA)
P	carbomer
P	disodium EDTA
H	benzophenone-4

3. Dermalogica Multi-Active Toner

S	water	
S	aloe (*Aloe barbadensis*) leaf juice	S: 6
H	butylene glycol	?: 2
P	lavender (*Lavandula angustifolia*) extract	P: 16
P	lemon balm (*Melissa officinalis*) extract	H: 4
P	mallow (*Malva sylvestris*) extract	
P	ivy (*Hedera helix*) extract	
P	cucumber (*Cucumis sativus*) extract	
P	elderberry (*Sambucus nigra*) flower extract	
P	arnica (*Arnica montana*) flower extract	
P	nettle (*Urtica* sp.) extract	
S	lavender (*Lavandula angustifolia*) essential oil	
S	lemon balm (*Melissa officinalis*) leaf extract essential oil	
P	sodium lactate	
P	sodium PCA	
S	sorbitol	
P	proline	
H	propylene glycol	
H	ricinoleth-40	
?	methyl gluceth-20	
P	polysorbate-20	
P	PEG-12 dimethicone	
?	polyquaternium-4	
P	disodium EDTA	
H	phenoxyethanol	

P	chlorphenesin
P	methylparaben
S	linalool

4. Banana Boat Aloe Vera with Vitamin E Sunscreen Lip Balm, SPF 30

Active ingredients

H	octyl dimethyl PABA	S: 7
H	octinoxate	?: 1
H	oxybenzone	P: 11
H	homosalate	H: 5
P	dimethicone	

Inactive ingredients

P	allantoin
P	aloe (*Aloe barbadensis*) leaf extract
S	beeswax (*Cera alba*)
P	butylparaben
S	coconut (*Cocos nucifera*) oil
S	candelilla (*Euphorbia antisyphilitica*) wax
H	fragrance
P	isopropylparaben
?	isocetyl alcohol
P	isobutylparaben
P	methylparaben
P	myristyl lactate
P	ozokerite
S	panthenol
P	petrolatum
S	castor (*Ricinus communis*) seed oil
P	silica
S	cocoa (*Theobroma cacao*) seed butter
S	tocopherol (vitamin E)

5. Tarte Vitamin-Infused Lipstick

P	octyldodecanol		**S: 13**
?	isohexadecane		**?: 10**
?	phenyl trimethicone		**S/P: 1**
?	trioctyldodecyl citrate		**P: 18**
P	glyceryl triacetyl hydroxystearate		**H: 1**
S	castor (*Ricinus communis*) seed oil		
S	candelilla (*Euphorbia antisyphilitica*)		
P	ozokerite		
?	octyldodecyl neopentanoate		
P	silica		
H	polyethylene		
S	jojoba (*Simmondsia chinensis*) seed oil		
P	VP/eicosene copolymer		
S	beeswax (*Cera alba*)		
S	carnauba (*Copernica cerifera*) wax		
P	kaolin		
?	polymethyl silsesquioxane		
?	tridecyl trimellitate		
S	meadowfoam (*Limnanthes alba*) seed oil		
?	cetyl ricinoleate		
?	phenylmethylsiloxane		
P	trimethylpentaphenyl trisiloxane		
S	tocopherol (vitamin E)		
S	ascorbyl palmitate		
P	butylated hydroxytoluene (BHT)		
S	shea (*Butyrospermum parkii*) butter		
P	magnesium carbonate		
P	grape (*Vitis vinifera*) seed extract		
?	dipotassium phosphate		
S	ascorbic acid (vitamin C)		
S	niacinamide (vitamin B-3)		
S	retinol (vitamin A) palmitate		
?	dicalcium sulfate dihydrate		

S	acai (*Euterpe oleracea*) fruit oil
P	green tea (*Camellia sinensis*) leaf extract
P	chamomile (*Chamomilla recutita*) extract

May contain

S/P	titanium dioxide
P	D&C Red 6
P	FD&C Yellow 5
P	FD&C Yellow 6
P	D&C Red 7
P	FD&C Blue 1
P	iron oxides

6. Dermablend Professional Cover Creme

Active ingredient

S/P	titanium dioxide	S: 2, ?: 1, S/P: 2, P: 9, H: 1

Inactive ingredients

P	mineral oil
H	talc
S	beeswax (*Cera alba*)
P	isopropyl palmitate
P	stearol stearate
P	kaolin
P	magnesium carbonate
S	carnauba (*Copernicia cerifera*) wax
P	allantoin
P	microcrystalline (*Cera microcristallina*) wax
?	lauroyl lysine

May contain

S/P	titanium dioxide
P	barium sulfate
P	iron oxides

7. Paula Dorf Eye Liner

P	cyclomethicone	S: 7
P	paraffin wax	?: 3
?	polybutene	P: 4
?	BIS diglyceryl polyacyladipate-2	H: 1
?	isocetyl alcohol	
S	meadowfoam (*Limnanthes alba*) seed oil	
S	sesame (*Sesamum indicum*) oil	
P	aloe vera (*Aloe barbadensis*) extract	
S	vitamin A	
H	PEG-8	
S	tocopherol (vitamin E)	
S	ascorbyl palmitate	
S	ascorbic acid (vitamin C)	
S	citric acid	
P	propylparaben	

8. Revlon ColorStay Mineral Eye Shadow

H	talc	S: 1
P	C12-15 alkyl benzoate	?: 4
?	caprylyl methicone	S/P: 9
P	cetearyl ethylhexanoate	P: 17
?	HDI/trimethylol hexyllactone crosspolymer	H: 2
?	diisostearyl malate	
P	magnesium aluminum silicate	
P	calcium aluminum borosilicate	
P	PPG-26-buteth-26	
P	ethylene/methacrylate copolymer	
*	zeolite	
*	mother-of-pearl	
*	topaz	
*	rose quartz	
P	silica	
?	isopropyl titanium triisostearate	
P	hydroxyethyl cellulose	

P	PEG-40 hydrogenated castor (*Ricinus communis*) oil
P	tetrasodium EDTA
H	phenoxyethanol
S	sorbic acid
P	butylated hydroxytoluene (BHT)
P	methylparaben
P	propylparaben
P	butylparaben

* no way to evaluate what form this is in or rate it (used in the table above)

May contain

S/P	mica
S/P	titanium dioxide
S/P	iron oxides
S/P	carmine
S/P	ultramarine
S/P	manganese violet
S/P	ferric ferrocyanide
S/P	bismuth oxychloride
S/P	chromium oxide green
P	FD&C Blue 1
P	FD&C Yellow 5
P	chromium hydroxide green

9. Max Factor Mascara

S	water	S:7
P	glyceryl stearate	?: 1
P	ammonium acrylates copolymer	S/P: 2
?	quaternium-18 hectorite	P: 15
H	propylene glycol	H: 4
S	stearic acid	
S	carnauba (*Copernica cerifera*) wax	
H	triethanolamine	
P	synthetic wax	
P	acrylates copolymer	

P	polyvinyl alcohol
P	propylene carbonate
S	lecithin
P	SD alcohol 40-B
P	sodium laureth sulfate
P	oleic acid
H	phenoxyethanol
P	ethylparaben
P	trisodium EDTA
P	dimethicone
S	xanthan gum
S	panthenol
H	benzyl alcohol
P	propylparaben
P	methylparaben
S	glycerin
S/P	iron oxides
S/P	titanium dioxide
P	ultramarine

10. Jean Naté Silkening Body Powder

H	talc	P: 2
P	kaolin	H: 2
P	magnesium carbonate	
H	fragrance	

11. Clean Ultimate Eau de Parfum

P	alcohol (denatured)	S: 1
H	fragrance	P: 5
S	water	H: 2
H	ethylhexyl methoxycinnamate	
P	butyl methoxy benzoyl methane	
P	PPG-26-buteth-26	
P	ethylhexyl salicylate	
P	PEG-40 hydrogenated castor (*Ricinus communis*) bean oil	

12. Tom's of Maine Spearmint Toothpaste

P	sodium fluoride	S: 3
P	sorbitol	P: 7
P	hydrated silica	
S	water	
P	natural flavors	
P	xylitol	
P	sodium lauryl sulfate	
P	zinc citrate trihydrate	
S	xanthan gum	
S	menthol	

13. Tom's of Maine Original Care Deodorant Stick: Unscented

H	propylene glycol	S: 5
S	water	P: 4
P	sodium stearate	H: 1
S	organic aloe vera (*Aloe barbadensis*) leaf juice	
S	witch hazel (*Hamamelis virginiana*) water	
P	glyceryl laurate	
P	chamomile (*Matricaria recutita*) aqueous extract	
P	hops (*Humulus lupulus*) extract	
S	ascorbic acid (vitamin C)	
S	organic lemongrass (*Cymbopogon* sp.) oil	

14. Dove Beauty Bar

?	sodium cocoyl isethionate	S: 5
S	stearic acid	?: 3
S	coconut acid oil	S/P: 1
S	sodium tallowate	P: 5
S	water	H: 2
?	sodium isethionate	
P	sodium stearate	
H	cocamidopropyl betaine	

?	sodium cocoate or palm kernelate
H	fragrance
S	sodium chloride
P	tetrasodium EDTA
P	trisodium etidronate
P	butylated hydroxytoluene (BHT)
S/P	titanium dioxide
P	sodium dodecyl benzene sulfonate

15. Dove Daily Moisture Therapy Shampoo

S	(aqua) water	S: 4
P	sodium laureth sulfate	?: 4
?	disodium lauryl sulfosuccinate	P: 21
H	cocamidopropyl betaine	H: 5
P	ammonium chloride	
P	glycol distearate	
S	glycerin	
H	fragrance	
?	dimethiconol	
P	cocamide MEA	
P	PEG-5 cocamide	
P	carbomer	
?	amodimethicone	
P	guar hydroxypropyltrimonium chloride	
H	triethanolamine (TEA) dodecylbenzene sulfonate	
P	tetrasodium EDTA	
H	DMDM hydantoin	
P	C11-15 pareth-7	
P	laureth-9	
P	ammonium xylenesulfonate	
H	PEG-45M	
P	trideceth-12	
P	PPG-9	

P	lysine hydrochloride
S	silk amino acids (alanine, glycine, serine, arginine, isoleucine, cystine, histidine, glutamic acid)
P	borage (*Borago officinalis*) extract
P	palmitic acid
S	stearic acid
P	linoleic acid
P	oleic acid
?	eicosenoic acid
P	methylchloroisothiazolinone
P	methylisothiazolinone
P	D&C Violet 2

16. Dove Daily Moisture Therapy Conditioner

S	water	S: 5
S	cetearyl alcohol	?: 2
P	cetrimonium chloride	P: 7
P	cyclopentasiloxane	H: 5
?	dimethiconol	
S	glycerin	
P	quaternium-18	
H	fragrance	
H	propylene glycol	
H	hydroxyethyl cellulose	
P	potassium chloride	
P	disodium EDTA	
H	DMDM hydantoin	
H	triethanolamine (TEA) dodecylbenzene sulfonate	
?	lysine HCl	
S	silk amino acids	
S	borage (*Borago officinalis*) seed oil	
P	methylchloroisothiazolinone	
P	methylisothiazolinone	

17. Dove Deep Moisture Facial Cream

Active ingredients

P	avobenzene	S: 3
P	ensulizole	?: 7
P	octinoxate	P: 15
H	octisalate	H: 6

Inactive ingredients

S	water
S	glycerin
?	isohexadecane
H	trolamine
?	sorbitan stearate
P	myristyl alcohol
P	cetyl alcohol
P	glyceryl dilaurate
P	stearyl alcohol
H	PEG-100 stearate
?	sucrose stearate
S	stearic acid
P	cholesterol
P	sodium PCA
P	linoleic acid
?	ceramide-3
?	ceramide-6-11
?	ceramide-1
?	phytosphingosine
P	sodium lactate
H	PEG-4 laurate
P	carbomer
H	fragrance
H	phenoxyethanol
P	methylparaben
P	propylparaben

P	disodium EDTA
P	iodopropynyl butylcarbamate

18. Body Benefits by Body Image Fragrant Bath Fizzy

S	sodium bicarbonate	S: 2
P	sodium carbonate	P: 7
P	sodium alkyl sulfate	H: 1
P	pentasodium triphospate	
S	citric acid	
H	fragrance	

May contain

P	FD&C Red 4
P	D&C Red 33
P	FD&C Yellow 5
P	FD&C Blue 1

19. Suave Kids Body Wash

S	water	S: 4
P	sodium laureth sulfate	?: 2
H	cocamidopropyl betaine	P: 5
?	cocamidopropyl hydroxysultaine	H: 5
S	sodium chloride	
S	glycerin	
H	propylene glycol	
H	fragrance	
?	polyquaternium-10	
P	tetrasodium EDTA	
H	PEG-150 distearate	
S	citric acid	
P	etidronic acid	
H	DMDM hydantoin	
P	iodopropynyl butylcarbamate	
P	D&C Red 33	

20. Sanctuary Spa Covent Garden Salt Scrub

S	sodium chloride	**S: 10**
P	mineral oil	**P: 8**
S	maris sal (sea salt)	**H: 1**
S	sweet almond (*Prunus amygdalus dulcis*) oil	
S	tocopherol (vitamin E) acetate	
S	wheat germ (*Triticum vulgare*) oil	
S	coconut (*Cocos nucifera*) oil	
H	perfume	
P	isopropyl myristate	
S	jojoba (*Simmondsia chinensis*) seed oil	
S	evening primrose (*Oenothera biennis*) oil	
P	hexyl cinnamal	
P	benzyl benzoate	
S	linalool	
S	limonene	
P	benzyl salicylate	
P	FD&C Yellow 33	
P	FD&C Red 23	
P	D&C Green 6	

21. Sanctuary Spa Covent Garden: Soothing Milk Bath

S	sodium chloride	**S: 8**
S	glucose syrup	**?: 3**
S	lactose	**P: 9**
S	African palm (*Elaeis guineensis*) kernel oil	**H: 1**
?	sodium cocyol isethionate	
?	sodium cocoyl glycinate	
P	magnesium sulfate heptahydrate	
P	kaolin	
S	avocado (*Persea americana*) oil	
S	evening primrose (*Oenothera biennis*) oil	
?	sodium caseinate	
H	perfume	

P	distilled monoglyceride
P	dipotassium phosphate
P	diacetyl tartaric acid ester of monoglycerides (DATEM)
P	silica
P	benzyl benzoate
P	benzyl salicylate
P	hexyl cinnamal
S	limonene
S	linalool

22. Neutrogena Body Oil

P	isopropyl myristate	S: 1
S	sesame (*Sesamum indicum*) seed oil	P: 4
P	PEG-40 sorbitan peroleate	H: 1
P	propylparaben	
P	butylated hydroxytoluene (BHT)	
H	fragrance	

23. Johnson's Baby Oil

P	mineral oil	S: 1
P	aloe (*Aloe barbadensis*) leaf extract	P: 2
H	fragrance	H: 1
S	tocopherol (vitamin E) acetate	

24. Origins Never a Dull Moment Skin-Brightening Face Polisher with Fruit Enzymes

S	water	S: 16
S	bitter orange (*Citrus aurantium amara*) flower water	?: 4
H	butylene glycol	P: 17
S	lecithin	H: 2
?	bethenyl betaine	
S	glycerin	
P	polysorbate-60	

P	propylene glycol stearate
P	polysorbate-20
?	sorbitan laurate
P	polysorbate-80
S	sodium chloride
P	papaya (*Carica papaya*) extract
S	buchu (*Barosma betulina*) leaf oil
S	grapefruit (*Citrus paradisi*) peel oil
S	eucalyptus (*Eucalytpus globulus*) leaf oil
S	Siberian fir (*Abies sibirica*) oil
S	mint (*Mentha arvensis*) leaf oil
S	bitter almond (*Prunus amygdalus amara*) kernel oil
S	limonene
S	apricot (*Prunus armeniaca regia*) shell powder
S	carnauba (*Copernicia cerfera*) wax
P	mango (*Mangifera indica*) extract
P	propylene glycol laurate
P	papain
P	carbomer
?	phosphorate phosphate
?	dimethyl isosorbide
S	potassium sorbate
P	sodium dehydroacetate
P	tetrasodium EDTA
H	phenoxyethanol
P	methylparaben
P	ethylparaben
P	propylparaben
P	butylparaben
P	isopropylparaben
P	isobutylparaben
S	essential oil

25. Aveeno Baby Soothing Relief Moisture Cream

S	water	S: 6
S	glycerin	P:13
P	petrolatum	H: 4
P	mineral oil	
P	cetyl alcohol	
P	dimethicone	
S	oat (*Avena sativa*) kernel flour	
P	carbomer	
H	ceteareth-6	
P	methylparaben	
S	sodium citrate	
P	tetrasodium EDTA	
P	stearyl alcohol	
H	benzalkonium chloride	
P	propylparaben	
P	ethylparaben	
P	PEG-25 soy sterol	
H	benzaldehyde	
S	hydrolyzed oats (*Avena sativa*)	
H	butylene glycol	
P	oat (*Avena sativa*) kernel extract	

May contain

P	sodium hydroxide
S	citric acid

26. Comodynes Makeup Remover with Oats

S	aqua (water)	S: 2
H	butylene glycol	?: 3
H	trideceth 9/PEG-5 octanoate	P: 9
S	glycerin	H: 5
P	oat (*Avena sativa*) extract	

?	sodium coceth sulfate
P	PEG-40 glyceryl cocoate
?	PPG-20 methyl glucose ether
H	propylene glycol
P	sodium methylparaben
P	sodium dehydroacetate
P	sorbic acid
P	tetrasodium EDTA
H	methyldibromo glutaronitrile (phenoxyethanol)
H	imidazolidinyl urea
P	trisodium EDTA
P	perfume
P	potassium phosphate
?	dipotassium phosphate

Just as a reminder, here are some things to keep in mind about how I rated certain ingredients:

◇ I have listed certain types of alcohol as potentially harmful. When it came to listing them, I vacillated between "safe" and "potentially harmful," since there is a lot of controversy in the research. On one hand, alcohol in large quantities is not good for you or your skin; on the other hand, it is great in small quantities for its antibacterial and preservative properties and for its use in the extraction of herbs. I find it safe, but in fairness to other ingredients with the same issues, I decided to rate it potentially harmful.

◇ Note on essential oils: I have them listed as most studies list them. They are, however, one of the natural ingredients with the highest amount of allergic reaction. Also, you will see ingredients on labels such as limonene, linalool, coumarin, and cintronellal. If you research these, you will find them listed as harmful in some studies. I listed them as safe. They are naturally occurring components of the essential oil. Use all essential oils with caution, keep away from mucus glands, and test a small area of your skin with the product before using.

Replacement Product Profile

- 25 products
- 308 safe (S)
- 4 not enough data (?)
- 0 harmful (H)

- 540 total ingredients
- 30 safe/potential (S/P)
- 18 potentially harmful (P)

1. Sumbody A–Z Face Cream (replaces Dermalogica Multivitamin Power Firm Face Cream)

S	water	S: 31
P	emulsifying wax	?: 1
S	stearic acid	S/P: 1
S	olive (*Olea europaea*) oil	P: 2
S	organic aloe (*Aloe barbadensis*) leaf juice	
S	vitamin A	
S	vitamin C ester	
S	wolfberry (*Lycium barbarum*), extracted in jojoba oil	
S	shiitake mushroom (*Lentinus edodes*), extracted in jojoba oil	
S	bamboo (*Bambusa* sp.), extracted in jojoba oil	
S	pomegranate (*Punica granatum*), extracted in jojoba oil	
S	rooibos (*Aspalathus linearis*), extracted in jojoba oil	
S	hibiscus (*Hibiscus sabdariffa*), extracted in jojoba oil	
S	asafetida (*Ferula foetida*), extracted in jojoba oil	
S	pear (*Pyrus communis*), extracted in jojoba oil	
S	white tea (*Camellia sinensis*)	
S	black tea (*Camellia sinensis*)	
S	green tea (*Camellia sinensis*)	
S	Himalayan raspberry root (*Rubus idaeus*), extracted in jojoba oil	
S	hazelnut (*Corylus avellana*)	
S	thale cress (*Arabidopsis thaliana*)	
S	seaweed (*Fucus* sp.)	
S	lecithin	
S	carrot (*Daucus carota sativa*) seed oil	
P	alpha-lipoic acid	
S	methylsulfonylmethane (MSM)	

S	wheat (*Triticum* sp.) amino acids
S	oat (*Avena sativa*) amino acids
S	vitamin E
S/P	zinc oxide
S	neem (*Melia azadirachta*) seed oil
S	rosemary (*Rosmarinus officinalis*) oil
S	black willow (*Salix nigra*) bark, extracted in jojoba oil
S	lichen (*Usnea barbata*), extracted in jojoba oil
?	potassium sorbate

2. Sumbody C Me Glow Face Cleanser: Normal/Dry (replaces Dermalogica Essential Cleansing Solution)

S	German chamomile (*Chamomila recutita*) flower water	S: 18
S	aloe (*Aloe barbadensis*) leaf juice	P: 1
P	emulsifying wax	
S	burdock (*Arctium lappa*), extracted in jojoba oil	
S	orrisroot (*Iris* sp.), extracted in jojoba oil	
S	evening primrose (*Oenothera biennis*) oil	
S	rose hip (*Rosa canina*) seed oil	
S	bilberry (*Vaccinium myrtillus*), extracted in jojoba oil	
S	sugarcane (*Saccharum officinarum*), extracted in jojoba oil	
S	sugar maple (*Acer saccharum*), extracted in jojoba oil	
S	orange (*Citrus sinensis*), extracted in jojoba oil	
S	lemon (*Citrus medica limonum*), extracted in jojoba oil	
S	rosemary (*Rosmarinus officinalis*) leaf, extracted in jojoba oil	
S	vitamin E	
S	xanthan gum	
S	neem (*Melia azadirachta*) seed oil	
S	black willow (*Salix nigra*) bark, extracted in jojoba oil	
S	lichen (*Usnea barbata*), extracted in jojoba oil	
S	calendula (*Calendula officinalis*), extracted in jojoba oil	

3. Sumbody Neroli Facial Toner (replaces Dermalogica Multi-Active Toner)

S	orange blossom water	**S: 11**
S	aloe (*Aloe barbadensis*) leaf juice	
S	witch hazel (*Hamamelis virginiana*) distillate	
S	bilberry (*Vaccinium myrtillus*), extracted in pure grain alcohol	
S	sugarcane (*Saccharum officinarum*), extracted in pure grain alcohol	
S	sugar maple (*Acer saccharum*), extracted in pure grain alcohol	
S	orange (*Citrus sinensis*), extracted in pure grain alcohol	
S	lemon (*Citrus medica limonum*), extracted in pure grain alcohol	
S	cranberry (*Vaccinium* sp.), extracted in pure grain alcohol	
S	tea tree (*Malaleuca alternifolia*) leaf oil in pure grain alcohol	
S	black willow (*Salix nigra*) bark, extracted in pure grain alcohol	

4. Sumbody Lucky Lips Lip Balm (replaces Banana Boat Aloe Vera with Vitamin E Sunscreen Lip Balm, SPF 30)

S	shea (*Butyrospermum parkii*) butter	**S: 8**
S	apricot (*Prunus armeniaca*) oil	
S	pistachio (*Pistacia vera*) oil	
S	beeswax	
S	castor (*Ricinus communis*) bean oil	
S	avocado (*Persea americana*) oil	
S	jojoba (*Simmondsia chinensis*) seed oil	
S	natural flavoring	

5. Sumbody Lipstick Mineral Makeup Starter Kit (replaces Tarte Vitamin-Infused Lipstick)

S/P	mica	**S: 23**
S/P	boron nitride	**S/P: 7**
S/P	titanium dioxide	
S/P	silica microspheres	
S/P	magnesium stearate	
S/P	pearl powder	

S/P	silk powder
S	shea (*Butyrospermum parkii*) butter
S	calendula (*Calendula officinalis*), extracted in jojoba oil
S	lavender (*Lavandula angustifolia*), extracted in jojoba oil
S	green tea (*Camellia sinensis*), extracted in jojoba oil
S	white tea (*Camellia sinensis*), extracted in jojoba oil
S	rooibos (*Aspalathus linearis*), extracted in jojoba oil
S	chamomile (*Chamomila recutita*), extracted in jojoba oil
S	licorice (*Glykyrrhiz glabra*) root, extracted in jojoba oil
S	horsetail (*Equisetum arvense*), extracted in jojoba oil
S	chestnut (*Castanea* sp.), extracted in jojoba oil
S	chrysanthemum (*Chrysanthemum* sp.), extracted in jojoba oil
S	burdock (*Arctium lappa*), extracted in jojoba oil
S	nettle (*Urtica dioica*) leaf, extracted in jojoba oil
S	rose (*Rosa canina*), extracted in jojoba oil
S	orrisroot (*Iris germanica*), extracted in jojoba oil
S	spirulina (*Arthrospira platensis*), extracted in jojoba oil
S	bladder wrack (*Fucus vesiculosus*), extracted in jojoba oil
S	kombu (*Laminaria japonica*), extracted in jojoba oil
S	shiitake mushroom (*Lentinus edodes*), extracted in jojoba oil
S	Irish moss (*Chondrus crispus*), extracted in jojoba oil
S	juniper (*Juniperus* sp.) berry, extracted in jojoba oil
S	kelp (*Ascophyllum nodosum*), extracted in jojoba oil
S	carrot (*Daucus carota sativa*) seed oil

6. Sumbody Mineral Makeup Foundation (in the Mineral Make-Up Starter Kit) (replaces Dermablend Professional Cover Crème)

S/P	mica	**S: 23**
S/P	boron nitride	**S/P: 7**
S/P	titanium dioxide	
S/P	silica microspheres	
S/P	magnesium stearate	
S/P	pearl powder	

S/P	silk powder
S	shea (*Butyrospermum parkii*) butter
S	calendula (*Calendula officinalis*), extracted in jojoba oil
S	lavender (*Lavandula angustifolia*), extracted in jojoba oil
S	green tea (*Camellia sinensis*), extracted in jojoba oil
S	white tea (*Camellia sinensis*), extracted in jojoba oil
S	rooibos (*Aspalathus linearis*), extracted in jojoba oil
S	chamomile (*Matricaria recutita*), extracted in jojoba oil
S	licorice (*Glykyrrhiza glabra*) root, extracted in jojoba oil
S	horsetail (*Equisetum arvense*), extracted in jojoba oil
S	chestnut (*Castanea* sp.), extracted in jojoba oil
S	chrysanthemum (*Chrysanthemum* sp.), extracted in jojoba oil
S	burdock (*Arctium lappa*), extracted in jojoba oil
S	nettle (*Urtica dioica*), extracted in jojoba oil
S	rose (*Rosa canina*), extracted in jojoba oil
S	orrisroot (*Iris germanica*), extracted in jojoba oil
S	spirulina (*Arthrospira* sp.), extracted in jojoba oil
S	bladder wrack (*Fucus vesiculosus*), extracted in jojoba oil
S	kombu (*Laminaria japonica*), extracted in jojoba oil
S	shiitake mushroom (*Lentinus edodes*), extracted in jojoba oil
S	Irish moss (*Chondrus crispus*), extracted in jojoba oil
S	juniper (*Juniperus communis*) berry, extracted in jojoba oil
S	kelp (*Ascophyllum nodosum*), extracted in jojoba oil
S	carrot (*Daucus carota sativa*) seed oil

7. Sumbody Eyeliner (in starter kit) (replaces Paula Dorf Eye Liner)

S/P	mica	S: 23
S/P	boron nitride	S/P: 7
S/P	titanium dioxide	
S/P	silica microspheres	
S/P	magnesium stearate	
S/P	pearl powder	
S/P	silk powder	

S	shea (*Butyrospermum parkii*) butter
S	calendula (*Calendula officinalis*), extracted in jojoba oil
S	lavender (*Lavandula angustifolia*), extracted in jojoba oil
S	green tea (*Camellia sinensis*), extracted in jojoba oil
S	white tea (*Camellia sinensis*), extracted in jojoba oil
S	rooibos (*Aspalathus linearis*), extracted in jojoba oil
S	chamomile (*Matricaria recutita*), extracted in jojoba oil
S	licorice (*Glykyrrhiza glabra*) root, extracted in jojoba oil
S	horsetail (*Equisetum arvense*), extracted in jojoba oil
S	chestnut (*Castanea* sp.), extracted in jojoba oil
S	chrysanthemum (*Chrysanthemum* sp.), extracted in jojoba oil
S	burdock (*Arctium lappa*), extracted in jojoba oil
S	nettle (*Urtica dioica*), extracted in jojoba oil
S	rose (*Rosa canina*), extracted in jojoba oil
S	orrisroot (*Iris germanica*), extracted in jojoba oil
S	spirulina (*Arthrospira* sp.), extracted in jojoba oil
S	bladder wrack (*Fucus vesiculosus*), extracted in jojoba oil
S	kombu (*Laminaria japonica*), extracted in jojoba oil
S	shiitake mushroom (*Lentinus edodes*), extracted in jojoba oil
S	Irish moss (*Chondrus crispus*), extracted in jojoba oil
S	juniper berry (*Juniperus communis*), extracted in jojoba oil
S	kelp (*Ascophyllum* sp.), extracted in jojoba oil
S	carrot (*Daucus carota sativa*) seed oil

8. Sumbody Eyeshadow (in starter kit) (replaces Revlon Colorstay Mineral Eye Shadow)

S/P	mica	S: 23
S/P	boron nitride	S/P: 7
S/P	titanium dioxide	
S/P	silica microsperes	
S/P	magnesium stearate	
S/P	pearl powder	
S/P	silk powder	

S	shea butter (_Butyrospermum parkii_)
S	calendula (_Calendula officinalis_), extracted in jojoba oil
S	lavender (_Lavandula angustifolia_), extracted in jojoba oil
S	green tea (_Camellia sinensis_), extracted in jojoba oil
S	white tea (_Camellia sinensis_), extracted in jojoba oil
S	rooibos (_Aspalathus linearis_), extracted in jojoba oil
S	chamomile (_Matricaria recutita_), extracted in jojoba oil
S	licorice (_Glykyrrhiza glabra_) root, extracted in jojoba oil
S	horsetail (_Equisetum arvense_), extracted in jojoba oil
S	chestnut (_Castanea_ sp.), extracted in jojoba oil
S	chrysanthemum (_Chrysanthemum_ sp.), extracted in jojoba oil
S	burdock (_Arctium lappa_) root, extracted in jojoba oil
S	nettle (_Urtica dioica_), extracted in jojoba oil
S	rose (_Rosa canina_), extracted in jojoba oil
S	orrisroot (_Iris germanica_), extracted in jojoba oil
S	spirulina (_Arthrospira_ sp.), extracted in jojoba oil
S	bladder wrack (_Fucus vesiculosus_), extracted in jojoba oil
S	kombu (_Laminaria japonica_), extracted in jojoba oil
S	shiitake mushroom (_Lentinus edodes_), extracted in jojoba oil
S	Irish moss (_Chondrus crispus_), extracted in jojoba oil
S	juniper (_Juniperus communis_) berry, extracted in jojoba oil
S	kelp (_Ascophyllum_ sp.), extracted in jojoba oil
S	carrot (_Daucus carota sativa_) seed oil

9. Musq Musqhave Mineral Mascara (replaces Max Factor Mascara)

S	water	S: 9
P	alcohol	S/P: 2
S	jojoba (_Simmondsia chinensis_) seed oil	P: 2
S	castor (_Ricinus communis_) bean oil	
S	carnauba (_Copernicia cerifera_) wax	
S	cetyl alcohol	
P	emulsifying wax NF	
S	glycerin	

S	gum arabic
S	stearic acid
S/P	mica
S/P	iron oxides
S	pomelo (*Citrus grandis*) seed extract

10. Sumbody Body Powder: Citrus (replaces Jean Naté Silkening Body Powder)

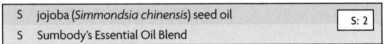

S	arrowroot (*Maranta arundinacea*) powder	**S: 4**
S	rice starch	
S	tapioca starch	
S	Sumbody's Essential Oil Blend	

11. Sumbody's Pure Sense Roll-On Perfume: Citrus Splash, Lavender, Ice Queen (replaces Clean Ultimate Eau de Parfum Spray)

S	jojoba (*Simmondsia chinensis*) seed oil	**S: 2**
S	Sumbody's Essential Oil Blend	

12. We did not switch Tom's Mint Toothpaste.

Since she is a single mother on a budget who recently bought several tubes of Tom's on sale, she did not want to throw out her current toothpaste. I gave her options for when she was finished with her current stock.

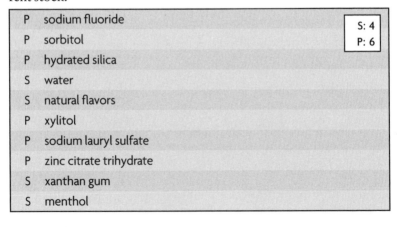

P	sodium fluoride	**S: 4**
P	sorbitol	**P: 6**
P	hydrated silica	
S	water	
S	natural flavors	
P	xylitol	
P	sodium lauryl sulfate	
P	zinc citrate trihydrate	
S	xanthan gum	
S	menthol	

13. Sumbody Be Fresh Body Deodorant (replaces Tom's Original Unscented Deodorant)

S	distilled water	**S: 5**
S	witch hazel (*Hamamelis virginiana*) distillate	**P: 1**
S	aloe vera (*Aloe barbadensis*) juice	
P	organic grape alcohol	
S	mineral salts	
S	Sumbody's Essential Oil Blend	

14. Sumbody Body Soap (replaces Dove bar soap)

S	olive (*Olea europaea*) oil	**S: 6**
S	coconut (*Cocos nucifera*) oil	
S	palm (*Elaeis* sp.) kernel oil	
S	safflower (*Carthamus tinctorius*) oil	
S	castor (*Ricinus communis*) bean oil	
S	Sumbody's Essential Oil Blend	

15. Chagrin Valley Soap & Craft Company Shampoo Bar: Babassu and Marsh Mallow (replaces Dove Moisturizing Shampoo)

S	saponified oils of an organic marsh mallow (*Althaea officinalis*) root	**S: 19**
S	grape (*Vitis vinifera*) seed	**P: 2**
S	avocado (*Persea americana*)	
S	babassu (*Orbignya oleifera*)	
S	coconut (*Cocos nucifera*)	
S	castor (*Ricinus communis*) bean	
S	palm (*Elaeis* sp.) kernel	
S	camellia (*Camellia sinensis*)	
S	jojoba (*Simmondsia chinensis*)	
P	wheat germ (*Triticum vulgare*) butter	
S	mango (*Mangifera indica*) butter	
S	walnut (*Juglans regia*)	
S	shea (*Butyrospermum parkii*) butter	

S	rice bran
S	marsh mallow (*Althaea officinalis*) root mucilage
S	organic aloe (*Aloe barbadensis*)
S	ylang-ylang (*Cananga odorata*) essential oil
S	lemon (*Citrus medica limonum*) essential oil
S	ginger (*Zingiber officinale*) essential oil
S	vitamin E oil
P	rosemary (*Rosmarinus officinalis*) oil extract

16. Sumbody Head First SumConditioner (replaces Dove Moisturizing Conditioner)

S	cetearyl alcohol	S: 11
P	glyceryl stearate	?: 1
S	macadamia (*Macadamia* sp.) nut oil	P: 1
S	cupuaçu (*Theobroma grandiflorum*) seed butter	
S	avocado (*Persea americana*) oil	
S	chrysanthemum (*Chrysanthemum* sp.)	
?	abyssine (*Alteromonas ferment*)	
S	acai (*Euterpe oleracea*)	
S	andiroba (*Carapa* sp.)	
S	copaiba balsam (*Copaifera officinalis*)	
S	olive (*Olea europaea*) oil	
S	sweet almond (*Prunus amygdalus dulcis*) oil	
S	Sumbody's Essential Oil Blend	

17. Sumbody DelightFULL Face Cream (replaces Dove Deep Moisture Facial Cream)

S	aloe (*Aloe barbadensis*) juice	S: 31
S	German chamomile (*Chamomila recutita*) flower water	P: 1
S	shea (*Butyrospermum parkii*) butter	
S	jojoba (*Simmondsia chinensis*) seed oil	
S	kosher vegetable glycerin	
S	cucumber (*Cucumis sativus*) fruit water	

P	emulsifying wax
S	vitamin C ester
S	green tea (*Camellia sinensis*), extracted in jojoba oil
S	nettle (*Urtica dioica*), extracted in jojoba oil
S	evening primrose (*Oenothera biennis*) oil
S	rose hip (*Rosa canina*) seed oil
S	carrot (*Daucus carota sativa*) seed oil
S	vitamin E
S	lecithin
S	vitamin A
S	xanthan gum
S	neem (*Melia azadirachta*) seed oil
S	cranberry (*Vaccinium macrocarpon*), extracted in jojoba oil
S	bilberry (*Vaccinium myrtillus*), extracted in jojoba oil
S	sugarcane (*Saccharum officinarum*), extracted in jojoba oil
S	sugar maple (*Acer saccharum*), extracted in jojoba oil
S	orange (*Citrus* sp.), extracted in jojoba oil
S	lemon (*Citrus medica limonum*), extracted in jojoba oil
S	Irish moss (*Chondrus crispus*), extracted in jojoba oil
S	birch (*Betula* sp.) bark, extracted in jojoba oil
S	orrisroot (*Iris germanica*) extract
S	rosemary leaf (*Rosmarinus officinalis*) extract
S	black willow (*Salix nigra*) bark extract
S	lichen (*Usnea barbata*) extract
S	myrrh essential oil
S	calendula (*Calendula officinalis*), extracted in jojoba oil

18. No replacement needed; eliminate fizzer. On a special occasion, use Sumbody Fizzer (replaces Body Benefits by Body Image Fragrant Bath Fizzy).

S	sodium bicarbonate	S: 3
S	citric acid	
S	Sumbody's Essential Oil Blend	

19. Sumbody Body Soap (see #14) (replaces Suave Kids Body Wash)

20. Sumbody Salt Scrub: Zen (replaces Sanctuary Spa Covent Garden Salt Scrub)

S	Pacific sea salt	S: 6
S	safflower (*Carthamus tinctorius*) seed oil	
S	pistachio (*Pistacia vera*) oil	
S	cocoa (*Theobroma cacao*) butter	
S	shea butter (*Butyrospermum parkii*)	
S	Sumbody's Essential Oil Blend	

21. Fresh or powdered milk with essential oils. For a special occasion, Sumbody Wholesum Bath Milk (replaces Sanctuary Spa Covent Garden: Soothing Milk Bath)

S	coconut (*Cocos nucifera*) milk	S: 6
S	whey	P: 1
S	milk	
S	buttermilk	
S	cream	
S	yogurt	
P	Sumbody's Scent Blend	

22. Sumbody Potion #9 Massage Oil (replaces Neutrogena Body Oil)

S	pistachio (*Pistachia vera*) oil	S: 13
S	apricot (*Prunus armeniaca*) oil	
S	jojoba (*Simmondsia chinensis*) seed oil	
S	safflower (*Carthamus tinctorius*) oils	
S	rose petals (*Rosa canina*)	
S	damiana (*Turnera aphrodisiaca*)	
S	alkanet (*Alkanna tinctoria*)	
S	jasmine (*Jasminum officinale*)	
S	clove (*Syzygium aromaticum*)	

S   vanilla (*Vanilla* sp.)

S   rose hip (*Rosa canina*)

S   cinnamon (*Cinnamomum zeylanicum*)

S   Sumbody's Essential Oil Blend

23. Eliminate Johnson's Baby Oil (Instead, use #22 above, Sumbody Potion #9 Massage Oil)

24. Sumbody Manna Facial Scrub (replaces Origins Never a Dull Moment Skin-Brightening Face Polisher with Fruit Enzymes)

S   honey   S: 9

S   Pacific sea salt

S   pistachio (*Pistacia vera*) oil

S   safflower (*Carthamus tinctorius*) seed oil

S   colloidal oats (*Avena sativa*)

S   avocado (*Persea americana*) oil

S   St. John's wort (*Hypericum perforatum*) oil

S   green tea (*Camellia sinensis*)

S   bee pollen

25. Sumbody Goat Milk Body Cream (replaces Aveeno Baby Soothing Relief Moisture Cream)

S   water   S: 21, ?: 1

S   xanthan gum

S   kosher vegetable glycerin

S   olive (*Olea europaea*) oil

S   stearic acid

S   coconut (*Cocos nucifera*) oil

S   sweet almond (*Prunus amygdalus dulcis*) oil

S   grape (*Vitis vinifera*) seed oil

S   avocado (*Persea americana*) oil

S   goat milk

S   rosemary (*Rosmarinus officinalis*) leaf, extracted in jojoba oil

S	vitamin A
S	vitamin C
S	vitamin E
S	witch hazel (*Hamamelis virginiana*) distillate
S	neem (*Melia azadirachta*) seed oil
S	chrysanthemum (*Chrysanthemum* sp.), extracted in jojoba oil
?	abyssine (*Alteromonas ferment*)
S	copaiba balsam (*Copaifera officinalis*)
S	andiroba (*Carapa guianensis*)
S	acai (*Euterpe oleracea*)
S	potassium sorbate

26. Sumbody Face Cream (see #1) or pure olive or safflower oil (replaces Comodynes Makeup Remover with Oats)

The Verdict

My goal with Barbara was not only to improve her skin and lessen her exposure to chemicals but also to save her money and improve her daughter's skin. The chemical-free makeover was successful on all counts.

Our first step was to reduce the number of products she was using. I also taught her many techniques for getting all of the benefit of body products without purchasing expensive specialty items—for example, rather than buying bath fizzers for regular use, saving them for special occasions and instead using bulk powdered milk and essential oil on a daily basis. Next, I eliminated her makeup-remover pads—they were toxic, expensive, and accelerating signs of aging. Instead, I told her to use oil she had in her house, such as olive, safflower, or almond oil. In an effort to be cost-conscious I decided to see if I could move her family away from liquid shampoo and move her to the most economical switch, shampoo bars. The switch worked—they all loved it. I replaced all of her products with chemical-free alternatives that gave her the results she was after and saved money. It was easy to replace her more expensive skin-care products and reduce costs, but what she didn't know was that the products she'd been using were so riddled with chemicals that they were part of her skin problems. Just getting her off of these products alone would have improved her skin.

One of her favorite swaps was the mineral makeup. I sent her a starter kit that included everything she used, except mascara, and that allowed her to blend her own colors. It provided a large array of colors as well as some fun. Both Barbara and her daughter loved the coverage, colors, versatility, and reduced cost. The price of the kit was not much more than that of the three compacts she was using from the drugstore, and she no longer had to buy eyeliner, lipstick, lip liner, and brow pencils—the Mineral Make-Up Starter Kit had it all.

With Barbara shifted to healthy and effective products, I moved on to her daughter. Even though she wasn't part of the makeover, I knew I could help. She had been suffering from worsening acne and all of the social disadvantages this meant for a sixth-grader. Already motivated to cure it, she diligently followed the regime I set out for her. Within several weeks, her acne was almost completely cleared. The line I gave her is one I have spent years formulating and tweaking. One former employee still writes me yearly letters to thank me for giving her self-confidence and restoring her social life; another, whose son had tried everything, found that these products were the only thing that ever worked. My clients and customers are awed by their acne-free skin.

Within the first week, Barbara's daughter noticed her skin quality beginning to improve. She was so thrilled that she shared her products with her mother. She also told me that her friends and family were commenting on how good she looked. I especially love this makeover because I helped a single mother on a tight budget save money, heal her and her daughter's skin, improve their self-esteem, eliminate chemicals, and reduce packaging waste.

In both makeovers, I did not reduce the amount of overall ingredients or products significantly. When asking people to make changes to their daily habits, I find it best to take it slow. It is a step-by-step process. First, to keep the person in their comfort zone, we change out the current product load and replace it with natural alternatives that will have the same or better results. Then, once they have acclimated and adjusted to that, I start the "reduction process," learning to use one product for multiple purposes. For example, Barbara can use the bar shampoo for body soap and choose between the body lotion and the massage oil. She can also choose between the A–Z Face Cream and the DelightFULL Face Cream. It is important to look at everything each of your products can do and limit your purchases.

PART IV

Recipes — and a Dash of Activism

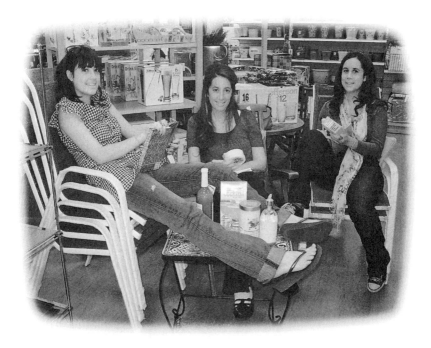

The Burnes Agency: Sleuthing out the chemicals in your body products at Marshalls

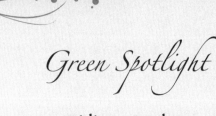

Green Spotlight

Didiayer Snyder,
Carpenter on Extreme Makeover:
Home Edition and Activist

"The way in which I live my daily life is an easy decision for me. We have one planet, one body, and one life. It is important for us to think about what we want to achieve while we are here. We have choices, and through these choices people can aspire to be the best they can be every day.

"This desire to be the best we can affects us on many levels. First, we need to love ourselves and treat our minds and bodies with respect. This means we need to be aware of the toxic substances we put into our body, onto our body, and surround ourselves with. Filling ourselves and our households with toxins when we have the knowledge to avoid them does not make sense.

"I have dedicated myself to a clean, green lifestyle for quite some time. Over the years my knowledge and information has grown, and with that I have changed many of my habits. I am extremely supportive of the work Deborah is doing and the message of this book. I think educating and empowering people is imperative. We should know what we are exposed to and what we are choosing.

"We think products' advertising images and slogans are what beauty is. Our frantic desire to be perfect makes us an easy target for products we do not need. We look at fancy ads and packaging and see a model who is sixteen, despite the product saying it will take wrinkles away. This simply is not true. We need to educate women and empower them on what really matters, and support that as a society, not oppress them with what they cannot change and what is not meaningful. We prey on their weaknesses, unhappy marriages, stress of raising children, and tell them that the way they look will fulfill them. The price is our health, both mentally and physically. In our yearning to be fulfilled, we put the emphasis on exterior boob jobs and manicures rather than directing it inward toward our beliefs and intrinsic worth as humans striving to be the best we can be.

"I have not escaped the desire to use products; it goes back to my childhood. My mother told me to put on lotion every morning and every evening, and I still do. My beauty secret is pure coconut oil. I get hydrated skin, it feels wonderful, and I am causing no harm to myself or the planet. Nor am I being sold fancy packaging or false promises. My real beauty secret is my heart. God blessed me with the way I look. I see myself as average, and what you are experiencing is my heart intention pouring out. You can see a beautiful woman who becomes ugly very quickly once you get to know her.

"All humans have these things in common—we are born and die, and we all desire to be accepted. For me, beauty begins and ends with self-acceptance and love. By giving, I become enriched. The more I give, the more I get and the more passionate I am about it. I love to inspire youths and teenagers because they are our future. I love to teach them what they are putting onto their skin. Beauty is one of the biggest changes we can make, both in how we feel about ourselves and how we affect our health. It effects what we put down our drains, onto our children, onto our pets, and onto our planet.

"Change starts organically. It starts with one voice—you talking to a neighbor, colleague, or friend. Change is something we can all be a part of. It is one more thing we can have in common as humans. We can all desire to be our best and create positive change for everyone.

"I do not need twenty different jars of expensive creams and lotions to feel fulfilled. I do not want to spend my life focusing on what is outside; I want to connect to what is inside. I want to build relationships that are sound and will last. I do not fear aging. I embrace it.

"I am so happy to be able to share my thoughts and feelings with others. I am so glad to be part of a larger shift and change. I believe wholeheartedly in Deborah's message and her way of educating people on caring for themselves. Beauty is self-love and acceptance. We need to be aware of how we treat ourselves and maintain our health and happiness so we can be of service to others. I appreciate Deborah's peek behind the world of cosmetics and beauty products, and I thank her for using her wisdom and knowledge to protect us, as well as our planet."

Chapter 17

Recipes

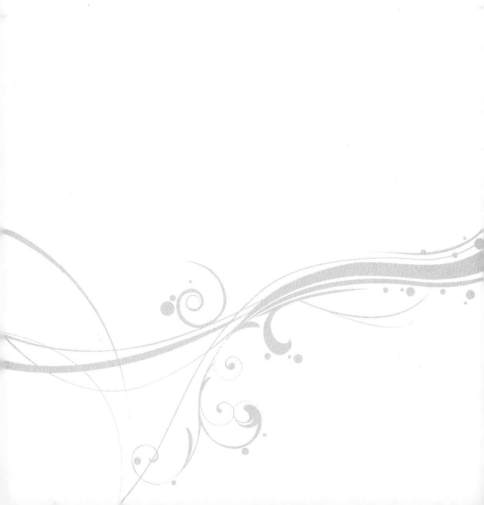

Making your own products at home is not only economical, fun, and simple, but it is also the safest, healthiest, and greenest choice of all. It is not always the most practical. In our already busy lives, fitting in one more thing can seem impossible. Over many years of experimenting I have come up with easy solutions for how you can squeeze in time for making a face mask or a salt scrub without disrupting your routine.

Growing up, my children loved to cook with me. From the time they could hold a knife, they were chopping, slicing, and dicing. Dinner became a time we all loved and embraced. We baked for fun. We also started to make bath products for ourselves and for gifts. This was a natural way to spend time with my children and get wonderful products. It was also a great teaching tool. We would measure, divide, and multiply, and learn about plants and herbs. We also had girls' night, where we would have a group over and make enough products for the month (you can freeze them), and at birthday parties we would make products. It can be a wonderful hobby with healthful benefits.

The following are a few tips for using the recipes below:

◇ Whenever possible, buy in bulk and buy organic.

◇ Fresh is best.

◇ Whenever possible, use glass for making and storing products. Recycle jelly, vinegar, mayonnaise, or any other type of glass jar you use.

◇ Store your products carefully. If you're making a dry product such as polishing grains, keep it away from moisture.

◇ If you're making a liquid, keep it in the refrigerator or freezer. Save time in the future by making extra and freezing it.

◇ Cleanliness is extremely important. You don't want hair or dirt from your hands in your gifts. You can either wash your hands well and sanitize with alcohol or wear gloves. Pull your hair back and wear a scarf or hairnet. Treat making products like you would preparing food: Apply the same rules for working with open cuts, wash your hands, and follow the other general rules of hygiene.

◇ Remember, when you wash your hands, you must dry them completely before continuing to make products.

The following are some easy recipes for products that are wonderful to use. After you get the basics, experiment and have fun with your own additions and twists; make them your own.

Have fun and enjoy!

Stress-Reducing Bath Salts

These salts take no time to make. You can make them in large amounts and store them for six months to a year, depending on whether or not you use olive oil. Olive oil makes the salts go from matte to shiny and adds moisture; leaving it out of the recipe greatly extends shelf life.

a large bowl	½ cup Epsom salt (optional, to relieve muscle tension)
a large spoon for mixing	2 drops lavender essential oil
a measuring cup	1 drop orange essential oil
a glass jar with lid (save old food jars, such as jelly jars or peanut butter jars)	1 teaspoon olive oil (optional— makes the salts go from matte to shiny, adds limited moisture)
1 cup pure sea salt (rock or granulated), not table salt	1 teaspoon lavender petals (optional)

Pour all of the salt into a large bowl. You can use any combination of pure sea salts and Epsom salts you choose. There are more and more of these on the market these days, making it fun to experiment. Kosher salt is a standard rock salt that is easy to find and wonderful to use (not all kosher salt is sea salt; check the box). If you are adding olive oil, mix the essential oils with the olive oil, then add to the salts; mix by hand or with a spoon. Sprinkle in the lavender petals. Pour the salts into a clean jar with a lid, and keep closed until ready to use. Essential oils will lose their scent over time if not in closed glass or a PET plastic jar.

Use 2 or more tablespoons per bath.

Wake-Up Bath Tea

a large bowl
a large spoon
a measuring cup
cheesecloth or a muslin bag
1 cup rosemary leaves, fresh or
    dried*

1 cup rose petals*
1 cup peppermint leaves*
1 drop each peppermint,
    eucalyptus, and rosemary
    essential oils
3 drops ginseng extract

Pour the rosemary, rose petals, and peppermint leaves into a large bowl. Using a spoon or your hands, gently toss, being careful not to crush the ingredients. Drop in the essential oils and ginseng extract and gently toss again. You can also mix by shaking in a Ziploc bag or a sealed plastic bowl. If you are using cheesecloth, cut two 6-inch × 6-inch squares and place one on top of the other. Put ½ cup of the "tea" mixture into the middle and draw all the sides and corners up, closing with a rubber band or thread. If using a muslin bag, fill it with ½ cup of the mixture and tie the bag shut. Place the bath tea in the tub while it is in the process of filling so the herbs have time to "brew" and infuse the bathwater.

* If you're using fresh herbs and petals, double the amount you place in the bag or cheesecloth.

The Ultimate Bathing Oil

a container to make and store oils
    in (an old food jar such as jelly
    jar or salad dressing jar)
a measuring cup
a measuring spoon

avocado, apricot, grape seed,
    almond, coconut, and/or
    olive oils
red turkey oil (note: this is not an
    animal product)
the essential oils of your choice

You can use any combination of the above oils. Avocado, apricot, and olive are richer; almond and coconut are lighter. Have fun finding a combination that works best for your skin. All these oils are so wonderful.

For every cup of oil, add ⅛ cup red turkey oil (this helps the oil suspend in your bathwater instead of only floating on top) and up to 10 drops of essential oils.

Please note: Using oils and butters in your bath makes surfaces slippery. Be careful when leaving your bath, and clean well after bathing.

Helpful hint: Keep baking soda near your bath and sprinkle it in after the water drains to absorb the excess oils; then wash the surfaces with soap.

Moisturizing Bath Fizzer

a large bowl	1 cup baking soda
a measuring cup	¼ cup citric acid
a measuring spoon	1 tablespoon powdered milk
a clean spray bottle of water	2 teaspoons cocoa butter
a flexible muffin pan (mold*)	5–20 drops essential oils

In a glass or metal bowl, mix the baking soda and citric acid; add the powdered milk. Melt the cocoa butter in a microwave until just melted but not scalding hot. Be very careful—heated butters can burn the skin. If the butter is too hot, let it cool a bit before using. When it is still melted and warm, mix with the dry ingredients, using a spoon or your hands. Add the essential oils and mix. The mixture should start to "come together" and feel slightly sticky. If needed, spray a *tiny* amount of water into the mixture, and press *firmly* into the muffin pan or molds. Let it dry overnight, then turn out of the mold.

* Teflon baking molds work great. They come in a muffin shape, and if you fill them ¾ of the way, they make a nice shape. Any hard plastic mold will work as well.

Butter Balm

a small mixing bowl	½ cup cocoa butter
a spoon	½ cup shea butter
a measuring cup	2 tablespoons apricot oil
a measuring spoon	essential oils

Melt the cocoa butter in a microwave until just melted but not scalding hot. Be very careful—heated butters can burn the skin. Add the shea butter. The heat from the cocoa butter should be enough to melt the shea. If it isn't, put the mixture in the microwave and cook it in 10-second intervals, waiting after each interval to give the shea a chance to melt, until it is completely melted. Add the apricot oil and blend well. You can add essential oils of your choice to create the scent level desired. Pour into a wide-mouth container or mold.

Body Oil

a small mixing bowl	½ cup jojoba oil
a spoon	1 cup safflower oil
a measuring cup	1 teaspoon carrot oil
a measuring spoon	1 teaspoon evening primrose oil
⅛ cup avocado oil	

Pour the oils into a glass jar with a lid. Close and shake well. Add essential oils of your choice to the scent level you desire.

Toothpaste

a small mixing bowl	3 teaspoons glycerin
a spoon	4–20 drops of flavoring (e.g., pep-
a measuring cup	permint extract)
a measuring spoon	1–3 drops of hydrogen peroxide
¼ cup arrowroot	for whitening (optional; check
1 teaspoon baking soda or	with your dentist)
orrisroot powder, or ½ tea-	
spoon of each	

In a small bowl, mix the arrowroot and orrisroot powder or baking soda. (I use orrisroot, but generations of people have been using baking soda with water as a toothpaste substitute. I would ask your dentist before using hydrogen peroxide or baking soda daily. In recent years there has been controversy over whether daily use is good for your enamel.) Add the glycerin and mix well. Add flavoring to taste.

Deodorant

a small mixing bowl
a spoon
a measuring cup
a measuring spoon
⅛ teaspoon fine-grain salt
3 teaspoons baking soda
3 teaspoons arrowroot

2 ounces beeswax
6 ounces safflower oil
3 drops rosemary essential oil
1 drop cedar essential oil
1 drop lavender essential oil
2 ounces carnauba wax

Please note: It is very hard to remove wax from utensils. I suggest finding something at a yard sale that you can use only for making personal-care products.

Put the salt in a mini-chopper or blender, and grind to a powder. Mix the salt, baking soda, and arrowroot in a small bowl, and set aside. Melt the beeswax and the carnauba wax over low heat or in a microwave (Caution: Heated waxes and oils can cause severe burns if they contact skin). Add all of the oils, mix with a metal spoon, and reheat if not completely liquefied. Add the dry ingredients to the wax-and-oil mixture (if the wax is not completely liquefied when you mix them, then heat again for a few seconds; the coolness of the powder mixture might start to solidify the waxes), and mix well.

Pour into molds, and chill in the refrigerator until solid.

Gentle Oat Face Cleanser for All Skin Types

a small mixing bowl
a spoon
a measuring cup
a measuring spoon
1 tablespoon shredded coconut
   (optional)

¼ cup cooked oats
1 tablespoon milk, soy milk, rice
   milk, or almond milk
1 tablespoon honey

Put the coconut in a food processor and pulse a few times. Combine the remaining ingredients in a small bowl, and mix well. Add the coconut and mix until completely incorporated.

Store in an airtight container. Use a dime-sized amount to cleanse your face. You can keep this in the refrigerator for a week, or freeze.

Almond Face Cleanser

a small mixing bowl
a spoon
a measuring cup
a measuring spoon
¼ cup finely ground almonds or almond meal

1 tablespoon milk
2 teaspoons licorice tea (use 1 tea bag and brew in ½ cup water; cool before using)
1 tablespoon brown rice syrup

In a small bowl, mix the almonds, milk, and tea. Add the brown rice syrup and mix until incorporated. Store in an airtight container.

Use a dime-sized amount to cleanse face. You can keep this in the refrigerator (in an air-tight container) for a week, or freeze.

Avocado Yogurt Face Mask

a small mixing bowl
a spoon
a measuring spoon
a mini food processor (you can still do this recipe without one—just mash very well!)

¼ banana, mashed
1 teaspoon mashed avocado
1 teaspoon plain Greek or regular yogurt
⅛ teaspoon brewer's yeast
⅛ teaspoon coconut milk

Place the banana and avocado in a mini food processor and purée. Add the remaining ingredients and mix well. Apply mask and leave on for 5 to 20 minutes, then rinse off. You can keep this in the refrigerator in an airtight sealed container for a week, or freeze in single-serving portions. This recipe makes two face masks.

Whipped Egg-White Face Mask

a small mixing bowl
a spoon
a measuring spoon
something with which to whip egg whites and cream
1 tablespoon whipping cream
1 egg white

1 tablespoon facial clay, such as French green clay (leave out if you can't find this item)
½ tablespoon rose jelly
½ tablespoon champagne (if you happen to have opened a bottle, save some and make this the next day; otherwise you can leave it out)

Whip the cream until stiff and set aside. Whip the egg whites until stiff, and set aside. Fold the clay, jelly, and champagne into the whipped cream, and blend well. Gently fold the cream mixture into the whipped egg white.

Alpha Hydroxy, Bioflavonoid Shower Face Mask/Cleanser/Scrub

You can use this as either a cleanser or a shower mask. Apply when you get into the shower and leave on, rinsing before you are done.

a small mixing bowl	1 tablespoon fruit jelly, any kind
a spoon	½ teaspoon citrus juice
a measuring spoon	1 teaspoon finely grated citrus rind
1 tablespoon honey	

Mix the honey and jelly in a small bowl; add the citrus rind and juice and stir well. Mix in the rind until incorporated. This will yield 6 different mask applications.

Note: The alpha hydroxy acids found in the fruit can cause skin sensitivity and redness in some people. Before using, apply a small amount to your inner wrist or a dime-sized amount on your cheek and leave on for 5 to 15 minutes to see if redness occurs.

Cucumber, Lemon, and Chamomile Toner

a small mixing bowl	1 cup apple cider vinegar
a spoon	(unfiltered organic works best)
a measuring cup	1 bag chamomile, green, white, and
a measuring spoon	or red (rooibos) tea*
1 cup sliced cucumber	3 cups distilled water
⅛ cup sliced lemon with rind	

In a jar with a lid (an old jam jar is perfect), combine the sliced cucumber, lemon, and vinegar. Chill in the refrigerator overnight.

Boil the water and then make the tea by letting it steep in the water until it cools. Remove the tea bag.

In a jar with a lid (an old jam jar is perfect), combine the sliced cucumber, lemon, cooled tea water, and vinegar. Chill in the refrigerator overnight.

Remove the cucumber and lemon slices from the water. Keep in the refrigerator.

For inflammation, redness, or irritated, sensitive skin, use chamomile tea.

For acne-prone skin, use red (rooibos) tea.

To combat wrinkles, use green or white tea.

Apply with a cotton ball or spray on the face as a mist. If the toner is too strong, or you don't like the smell of the vinegar, dilute it by adding more tea water. If you don't have a problem with a 25/75 vinegar/water ratio, it is the best. Apple cider vinegar is so wonderful for your skin. It restores pH; contains vitamins C, E, A, B-2, B-6, and P, as well as beta-carotene and alpha hydroxy acids; relieves sunburn; and reduces age spots. It also acts as an antiseptic, fighting viruses, bacteria, and yeast that can cause acne and infection.

This toner can be frozen in ice trays and used on hot days to cool down, tighten pores, and diminish blemishes.

Vitamin C Bioflavonoid Face Tea

High in vitamin C and bioflavonoids, this tea can be used as a face rinse/splash after washing, as a toner, or as a face mist (place in a misting bottle and spray on your face whenever you want); you can freeze it in ice trays and use it on hot days to cool down, tighten pores, and diminish blemishes.

a small mixing bowl	½ cup boiling water
a spoon	4 fresh rose hips, diced, or 1 bag
a measuring cup	rose-hip tea
a measuring spoon	2 teaspoons grated citrus rind

Steep the rose hips or tea in ½ cup lightly boiling water for 15 minutes. Add the grated citrus rind and set aside for another 15 minutes. Pour into a jar with a lid, seal, and refrigerate overnight. Strain the mixture the next day, and it is ready to use. Store in the refrigerator.

Brown Rice Face Exfoliant

a small mixing bowl
a spoon
a measuring cup
a measuring spoon
1 tablespoon brown rice flour

½ tablespoon finely ground almonds or almond meal
milk (soy, rice, almond, or dairy),
enough to make a paste

In a small bowl, combine the rice flour with the ground almonds, and mix well.

When you're ready to use, make a paste with milk or water, and wash your face with it, and rinse well.

Body Scrub

When choosing an oil, remember that different oils have different properties; some, such as olive, apricot, and avocado, are heavier; pistachio, safflower, and canola are lighter. Our Body Oil recipe (see page 276) makes a wonderful base for this scrub. Choose oils that feel the best on your skin.

For add-ins, be creative and have fun. You can use fresh milks, fruit purées, honey, vinegar, or champagne. The possibilities are un-limited.

a small mixing bowl
a spoon
a measuring cup
a measuring spoon
1 cup sea salt or sugar

enough oil (see above) to saturate
the salt
10–15 drops of your favorite essential oils
add-ins of your choice

In a medium-sized bowl, mix all the ingredients, using your hands, until well blended. If you use fresh ingredients, keep the mixture in a closed container in the refrigerator. Discard any unused scrub after a week. Without fresh ingredients, the scrub will last in a sealed con-tainer in your bathroom for approximately four to eight months or until the oils go rancid.

Hair Vinegar

This will restore pH, eliminate product buildup, close cuticles, and leave your hair shiny, smooth, and easy to manage and style.

a small mixing bowl	2 cups water (or 1 cup water and
a spoon	1½ cup beer)
a measuring cup	½ cup mixed herbs of choice (see
a measuring spoon	below)
	3 tablespoons apple cider vinegar

In a small pot, boil the water. Add the herbs, cover the pot, and let simmer for 15 minutes. Remove from heat, set aside, and let cool for one hour. Strain and add the apple cider vinegar.

Use the same day or keep in the refrigerator for up to a week. You can increase the recipe and keep any unused rinse in refrigerator as well.

Experiment by using 1½ cup of beer and 1 cup water. Do not boil the beer, but instead add it to the water and herb mixture after simmering.

After shampooing, apply the vinegar to your scalp and hair; leave on as long as you like, avoiding eye contact. You can either rinse with fresh water or leave it in your hair. The vinegar smell will dissipate shortly after your shower. The benefits are well worth the scent.

For all types of hair: rosemary, peppermint, calendula, parsley, nettle

For brittle, dry hair: horsetail, marigold, sage

For color-treated hair: nettle

For oily hair: lavender, tea tree oil, thyme, yarrow

For dandruff: tea tree oil, burdock, lavender, plantain, nettles. The acids and enzymes in apple cider vinegar kill bacteria that cause dandruff. You can increase the amount of vinegar as much as you like and leave it on your hair for a half hour.

To bring out natural highlights or to lighten: chamomile, marigold

To bring out natural dark highlights: sage, rosemary, parsley

Bath Vinegar

a small mixing bowl
a spoon
a measuring cup
a measuring spoon

1 cup apple cider vinegar
⅛ cup rice wine vinegar
herbs of your choice

You can add herbs and follow the hair vinegar recipe (see above) for infusing the herbs in the vinegar. The blend will restore pH, soothe itchy, brittle skin, cleanse, and remove dead skin cells.

Additional add-ins:

For dry skin: aloe vera juice, chamomile, oats, rose petals/hips
For oily skin: lavender, rosemary, citrus peel, sage

Hair Mask

a small mixing bowl
a spoon
a measuring cup
a measuring spoon
1 tablespoon banana

⅛ teaspoon honey
⅛ teaspoon lethicin
1½ tablespoons yogurt
1 teaspoon rice milk
1 teaspoon soy milk

Put all the ingredients into a blender. Blend to the consistency of a smoothie and continue blending a little longer. Use immediately.

There are two ways you can apply the mask. If you use leave-in products or have product buildup on your hair, wash first, towel dry, then apply. Otherwise apply to dry hair. Put a shower cap or plastic bag around your hair, and leave on for ½ hour. Rinse well, then shampoo.

After learning to make this basic mask, you can experiment and create new masks. Consistency is the key. Too runny and it is a drippy mess, too thick and pasty, and it is a nightmare to get out.

Also, try a beer rinse before your put the mask on your hair. Pour one-half of a can on dry hair; do not rinse out. Put the mask on over it. Beer is wonderful for adding bounce and shine and making hair fuller.

Add-ins:

For all hair types: egg, milk, mashed avocado

For oily hair: a combination of ⅛ teaspoon jojoba oil and ⅛ teaspoon wheat germ oil

For dry hair: a combination of ¼–½ teaspoon olive oil, ¼–½ teaspoon melted shea butter, and ¼–½ teaspoon jojoba oil

Gift Ideas, Holiday Themes

Since we are big bakers in my family, our friends, family, and neighbors are used to receiving our baked goods for every occasion. My girls brought cookies, cakes, and pastry to every school event. Somewhere along the line, we started cooking up bath concoctions instead of consumable goodies, and everyone loved them. For parties, birthdays, and teacher gifts, our treats were in high demand. But beware: When you start to give your loved ones your homemade products, they get hooked, and it is hard to keep the supply up with the demand. People will expect these homemade products, and they won't be shy about letting you know this when holidays, birthdays, and special events roll around.

Have Fun and Mix It Up

Bath products make the perfect holiday gift for everyone on your list. Pick a theme, such as "stress-free holidays," "beach paradise," "flower bouquet," or "Zen temple," and make an array of products with a scent that matches your theme. Fill a basket with bath salts, scrubs, body oil, and fizzers. Give them all names. For the stress-reducing gift, you can call a product "Give Me a Break" or "Letting Go." Attach cute stickers to the bottles and bags. (You can buy blank labels at any office-supply store.) Add a story about how you want to help all of your loved one survive holiday madness with your stress-reducing survival kit. There are countless themes, and you can change them every year. Everyone will be waiting to see what your new theme will be.

You can also make boy/girl gift packs and keep them handy for birthday gifts. Try a "birthday party" theme. You can make a "birthday cake" scrub with vanilla and chocolate extract and a touch of orange essential oil for scent; confetti fizzer with sprinkles (use the same ones you would eat); or bath salt with everything "party" in it (for an adult, use a little vodka for fun; for a child, use sprinkles, sugar instead of salt, etc.).

These custom treats also make wonderful wedding favors. At Sumbody, we make custom products for the bride and groom to give out as favors on their wedding day. We have them tell us their favorite scents or what they love to use. For example, the bride might love vanilla and anything that is relaxing, while the groom loves mint and soaks to alleviate muscle tension. We then make products that combine both of their loves, such as vanilla-mint, stress-reducing body scrub and muscle-ache-relieving bath salts. We make tiny sizes, put together adorable gift sets, and write a story about how the bride and groom met and how this represents the beginning of their lives together. Everyone loves this. To the bride and groom, it is personal, special, and different. And guests love receiving something they can really use, something beyond the usual almond candy or bubbles. Brides will adore you.

These gifts are also perfect for bridal showers, at teen pampering parties, as hostess thank-you gifts, and as dinner-party gift bags.

At Sumbody, we sell product-making kits that you can do as a group at a bridal shower or teen party or use by yourself. But you don't need a kit to have fun. You would be surprised to see what you can find close to home. Drugstores carry mason jars, which are wonderful for packaging, since everyone can reuse them (we drink out of them at my house). Craft stores, such as Michael's, sell glass jars and fun wrapping supplies; Wal-Mart and cake-decorating stores have supplies for wrapping and filling. Health-food stores usually sell essential oils, or you can order them online. With a little looking, you can probably find what you need close to home.

Chapter 18

What You Can Do to Help Tighten the Safety Standards for Beauty Products

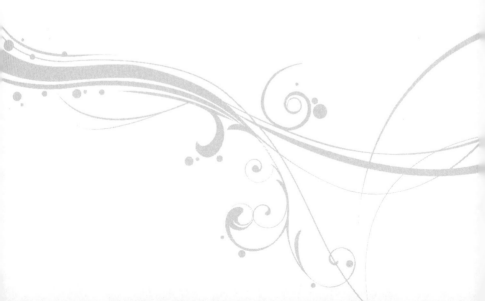

There is a lot you can do to improve safety standards for the beauty and health products you use every day. Look over the list below and choose to do a minimum of three things from the list this week—and you will start making a difference.

◇ Write a letter to Congress! Be a part of the nationwide campaign to stop untruthful label claims and increase transparency in the cosmetic industry. It is easy—just fill out this template and mail it to your congressperson:

Dear Member of Congress:

I strongly support the campaign to mandate truly safe cosmetics and urge the following policy implementations:

- sufficient documentation and testing to prove that each ingredient is nontoxic and not harmful before chemicals become available for use in personal-care products
- stringent federally regulated guidelines for what can and cannot be used in personal-care products
- mandatory label warnings of known potential adverse health effects until the chemicals are fully tested and/or eliminated from the market

Sincerely,

_____

First name, Last name

_____

E-mail

_____

Zip/postal code

◇ Support companies that list all their ingredients without tricks, such as "derived from" or "in a base of," and companies that will readily answer any questions or concerns.

◇ Expose your friends and family to healthful choices. Give body-care products for gifts. Everyone loves them, and by choosing alternative products you will be exposing others to healthy habits.

◇ Teach your children while they are young. Does a baby really need ten products a day? Limit your use; start them out with healthful products and a knowledge of what's being used and why.

◇ Look for healthful alternatives that work. Companies using all that science and nature have to offer, combined with beauty tips from around the world, have created wonderful products that yield truly effective results.

◇ Look for products that use food-grade ingredients.

◇ If you have questions about what's in a product, don't take "I don't know" or "It's all good" for an answer. If you suspect something is not right, dig until you find the answer.

◇ If a company makes it hard to find the answer, move on. We should not have to invest hours of research to find out what's in our products. The onus should be on the manufacturer to inform and disclose to consumers, not on the consumer to play detective.

◇ Consult the important and thorough research being done by many organizations—you just have to know where to look and how to use what you find. One of the most impressive resources I found was the American Cancer Society (1-800-ACS-2345). When I called and asked if I could get a list of known carcinogens used in the cosmetic industry, not only was the person I spoke to more than willing to help answer my questions, but he also e-mailed me a compendium of all known human carcinogens based on research done and/or reviewed by the ACS. In less than five minutes, I was given complete access to the forefront of medical research being performed in our country. Known carcinogens that are used in cosmetics include ethylene oxide, formaldehyde, and mineral oil, to name just a few. While I was on the phone, I also inquired about parabens. The ACS rep told me that there have been studies that have shown parabens in breast cancer tumors, but there have not been enough studies done to prove that the parabens caused the cancer, and he informed me that the ACS will perform further studies. This means you are getting the real deal—if the ACS says something is carcinogenic, you can be sure there is research to back it up. One word of caution: If you see an ingredient on the list of carcinogenic substances, be sure to look up its synonyms as well. Often, consumers are fooled into buying a product that contains an ingredient they are not comfortable using because it is hiding under a different name. To make sure this doesn't happen to you, go to http://householdproducts.nlm.nih.gov/index.htm and search for the ingredient in question—it will provide you with all the synonyms.

◇ Be satisfied with ingredients that exist and that we know are good. We have everything we need to make effective skin-care products, yet still we keep searching for the next "miracle" ingredient. If we could be satisfied with the options we have, we would severely reduce both the environmental impact of creating these ingredients and our exposure to harmful chemicals. We have become a society of constant stimulation and disposability. We expect everything to be fast, exciting, new, and attractive, and we assume that if it isn't, it must be boring and ineffective. Children can't cope without the speedy rate at which scenes change in Sesame Street, and some adults have taken to disposing of socks and underwear after one use; we use and toss plastic bags, water bottles, and unnecessary packing of all kinds. Our short attention span fuels the production of more and more ingredients, most of which are harmful, with the same properties as those that already exist. If we can be satisfied with the ingredients that exist, there will be less pressure on manufacturers to keep producing new ingredients. This is one way we can influence the industry to conform to our standards, and in doing so, reduce harm.

◇ Stop polluting ourselves and our environment. Why can we see that we are polluting the environment but not correlate that to ourselves? If we see trees dying, the earth slowly being destroyed, and landfills overflowing, how can we not see that these same chemicals that are harming the environment are having an effect on our health?

If we had violent stomach cramps or broke out in a rash every time we applied chemical products to our skin, we would throw them in the trash immediately and probably call the company to demand a refund, or more. There would be petitions, and companies and manufacturers would have to start taking some responsibility. As it is, we don't see these immediate symptoms. Instead we see long-term health effects and complications that develop over time and are much more dangerous than a one-time painful rash. Whether we do not connect these problems to our beauty products or are in denial, the fact is that just like the earth, our bodies are being harmed by the pervasive use of chemicals on our skin. We have Save the Earth petitions and cleanup days, but do we see cleanup days for humans? Do we institute a national Save the Humans Day? No, because we do not recognize the degeneration that is slowly taking place within our species. We are conditioned from infancy to trust certain brands and chemicals. We use them for cleaning our dishes, brushing our teeth, washing our clothes, scrubbing our countertops, and innumerable other mundane tasks. This early acculturation to synthetics renders us nearly incapable of turning against them, even as they harm our bodies and our children.

It is time we realize the true capacity of these chemicals to harm us and begin to make educated, well-informed choices. It is not that we have to eliminate everything chemical from our lives, but rather that we should not include anything in our regimen unless we fully understand it and make a conscious and informed decision to use it. It took time for us to see the effects of these chemicals and the production of these chemicals on the environment—let's not wait to see them in ourselves.

◇ Read your labels and educate yourself on what is inside of a product. Knowledge is power. Take the label test. Go to your bathroom and look at the products you and your loved ones are using, even if they are labeled "natural" or "organic." If you do not clearly understand every ingredient or suspect that the product contains toxic chemicals, stop using it. Find out about every single element in the product. With convenient access to the Internet, we have a world of information at our fingertips. If you find a product is toxic, dispose of it at a household toxic waste site and choose clean and safe products in the future. The real ones are few and far between, but they do exist.

◇ Speak with your wallet, since manufacturers listen. But beware of the sneaky tricks they play with you in the process. With the growing public concern over the paraben family of preservatives (methyl, butyl, propyl) in light of the growing scientific evidence of severe adverse health effects, the manufacturers are one step ahead and have a solution. Their clever response is to remove the parabens and promote "new" and "paraben-free" products. Sounds great, and one would almost think that they are "cleaning up their act." One would wish and hope this were in fact the truth. The truth, however, is that they are hooking you by calming your fears of parabens (a little knowledge can be a harmful thing) and replacing the parabens with yet another toxic chemical preservative that the public is not aware of...YET. All we see is what we want. We see paraben-free, sodium lauryl sulfate-free, or propylene glycol-free and we're hooked. We believe, once again, that the product in question is natural and good for us.

◇ Be your own advocate for health and safety; there is no one else looking out for your welfare. We live in a society driven by the bottom line, where money speaks louder then human welfare. In 1999 scientists at Stanford released a study showing the absorption rate of chemicals via personal-care products. They found that they could deliver an effective dose of a vaccine in a shower with just one shampooing. The vaccine was absorbed into the bloodstream through the hair follicles on unshaven, unbroken skin. If we can administer a large enough dose of a vaccine in a single shampooing, what are all the chemicals in our daily "cleaning and beautifying" routine doing to our health? We are, in essence, feeding these cosmetic chemicals to our brain, organs, and nervous system every day. We have become a nation that is feeding off the "ultimate junk food," the ultimate poison. Our bodies were not made to process all these toxins and chemicals. We have put our systems on overdrive and they can no longer sustain the personal attack, the personal pollution. Our cup is full; the state of our personal health is overflowing with adverse issues. There is no way for us to be at our peak of health when we are constantly attacking ourselves with a vast array of man-made chemicals.

Did You Know?

The chemicals industry claims the substances it produces are adequately controlled and do not pollute the environment. However, detailed scientific studies have found man-made toxic chemicals present in the bodies of polar bears, in Alpine lakes, and in indigenous populations thousands of kilometres from the source of these chemicals. Our own scientific investigations have detected toxic chemicals in our homes, in our blood, in rainwater. Unborn infants are exposed to many man-made pollutants while still in the womb.

— Green Peace

◇ According to a report commissioned jointly by Greenpeace International, Greenpeace Netherlands, and WWF-UK, hazardous chemicals are clearly present in maternal and umbilical cord blood samples. http://reach.org.my/index.php?option=com_content&task=view&id=360&Itemid=68

◇ Under the authority of the Fair Packaging and Labeling Act (FPLA), the FDA requires an ingredient declaration on the cosmetic products sold at the retail level to consumers. However, the regulations do not require the listing of the individual fragrance ingredients and the FPLA does not apply to products used exclusively by professionals (e.g., products used in spas and salons). Additionally, the regulations only specify that the listing has to appear "on the cosmetic product," and I have seen companies use accordion-style labels (the ingredients are technically on the product) so that you cannot read the ingredients until you purchase the product.

◇ L'Oreal has gobbled up the Pureology brand. This luxury American brand is sold through professional hairdressers and is known for its range of sulfate-free shampoos. Unfortunately, it is now gaining in popularity since it has the power of L'Oreal behind it, but its ingredients are not safe or natural at all. This is an example of things to be aware of and watch out for.

◇ According to the marketing information company NPD Group, sales of prestige skin-care products in U.S. department stores alone reached $2.1 billion in 2004, up 17 percent from 2000.

◇ If you want to be healthy, look to your skin to tell you how you are doing at achieving it. The state of your skin is the ultimate reflection of how healthy you are on the inside.

◇ In an analysis of twenty breast tumors, researchers found high concentrations of para-hydroxybenzoic acids (parabens) in eighteen samples. Parabens can mimic the hormone estrogen, which is known to play a role in the development of breast cancers. The preservatives are used in many cosmetics and some foods to increase their shelf life. "From this research it is not possible to say whether parabens actually caused these tumours, but they may certainly be associated with the overall rise in breast cancer cases," says Philip Harvey, an editor of the *Journal of Applied Toxicology*, which published the research.

◇ 12.2 million adults are exposed to known or probable human carcinogens through daily use of personal-care products.

◇ 4.3 million women are exposed daily to toxic ingredients linked to fertility impairment and fetal development problems.

(cont'd.)

◇ Twenty percent of all adults are exposed daily to the top seven carcinogens commonly found in personal-care products: hydroquinone, ethylene, dioxide, 1,4-dioxane, formaldehyde, nitrosamines, PAHs, and acrylamide.

◇ One of the top four revenue-grossing products made in the United States is chemicals, which includes cosmetic chemicals. The industry was worth 250 billion dollars in 2007 (up from 174 billion dollars in 2002), at which time it was employing 830,000 Americans.

◇ In 2004 the Environmental Working Group (EWG) stated that 99.9 percent of the 7,500 personal-care products they analyzed contained one or more ingredients never studied for safety by the Cosmetic Ingredient Review (CIR).

According to an independent (unpublished) survey of 172 participants by the manufacturer of Ocean Pure Cleansing Spray (Page & Ridout 2006; contact the company for more information on their study):

◇ 34 percent of consumers read the labels on baby products.

◇ 90 percent of consumers read the labels on food products.

◇ 80 percent of consumers bought their baby products from major supermarkets.

Seeing this peaked my curiosity, so we conducted our own survey at our retail stores. We asked five-hundred people, and although we expected that our customers would be even more savvy and educated than the average person, we came up with figures that were within 2 percent of theirs.

Who is protecting our children? It is time to start taking notice.

Resources, Ingredients, References

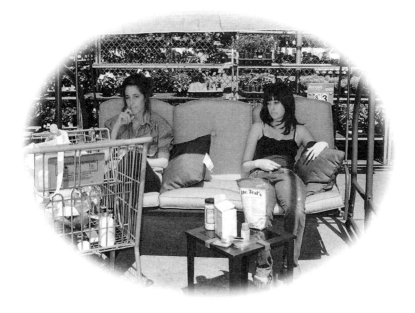

Worn out after a hard day's work as label detectives, Mica and I catch a quick break in the Home and Garden section of Cost Plus

Appendix A:
Resources for Research at Home

http://householdproducts.nlm.nih.gov/index.htm
Information on both household and personal-care products, as well as MSDS and other information on chemicals. Learn more about what's in these products, potential health effects, and safety and handling.

http://toxnet.nlm.nih.gov
Toxicology, environmental-health, and chemical databases, as well as other information resources from the Toxicology and Environmental Health Information Program.

www.ejnet.org/toxics
A website focusing on environmental health, children's environmental health, pesticides, and toxic chemicals. Contains a database of information on toxic pollution and provides results from pollution mapping projects.

www.safecosmetics.org
A coalition of U.S. health and environmental nonprofit groups working to promote nontoxic personal-care products. Includes news, articles, FDA regulations, and more.

www.bcaction.org
Breast Cancer Action is a national grassroots education and advocacy organization. This website includes information, articles, and updates on chemicals that can contribute to cancer, including those we are exposed to in personal-care products.

www.ewg.org
The Environmental Working Group (EWG) works to protect children and kids from toxic chemicals in our food, water, air, and the products we use. The website contains resources for consumer products and chemical safety, research, and articles.

www.cosmeticsdatabase.com
Skin Deep, The Environmental Working Group's searchable database of toxic ingredients in cosmetic and personal-care products, is the first comprehensive look at cosmetic chemicals and products and their known toxic effects on our health.

www.organicconsumers.org
Contains information such as The Organic Consumers Association and GreenPeople.org's huge Greenpeople Directory of green and organic businesses; updates on chemicals, organic standards, and the fair trade movement.

www.breastcancer.org
A nonprofit website that includes pertinent information on breast cancer, chemicals, and cancer in general.

www.cir-safety.org
The Cosmetic Ingredient Review thoroughly reviews and assesses the safety of ingredients used in cosmetics in an open, unbiased, and expert manner, and publishes the results in the peer-reviewed scientific literature.

www.personalcarecouncil.org
Contains a review of cosmetic ingredients.

www.cosmeticsinfo.org
A source for safety information about cosmetic and personal-care products, their ingredients, and how they are tested and regulated. You may not agree with their safety assessments, but the site does a wonderful job of explaining what an ingredient is.

www.pubmed.gov
Use to look up studies on chemicals.

http://hazmap.nlm.nih.gov
Haz-Map is an occupational toxicology database designed to link jobs to hazardous job tasks that are linked to occupational diseases and their symptoms. It is a relational database of chemicals, jobs, and diseases.

www.atsdr.cdc.gov
The Agency for Toxic Substances and Disease Registry (ATSDR) serves the public by using the best science, taking responsive public health actions, and providing trusted health information to prevent harmful exposures and diseases related to toxic substances.

www.scorecard.org
Find environmental information about your community: Learn how bad

the pollution is, where the toxic chemicals come from, and what the health risks are.

www.sciencedirect.com
An information source for scientific, technical, and medical research. A subscription is required for some sections.

www.environmentialchemistry.com
Provides environmental, chemistry, and hazardous-materials news, information, and resources.

www.osha.gov
The Occupational Safety and Health Administration (OSHA) website. OSHA's website contains information on how to protect yourself from chemical exposure at your workplace.

www.cdc.gov
The website for the Centers for Disease Control and Prevention (CDC) contains information on health and safety topics, including chemicals in personal-care products and reported poisonings from them.

www.cdc.gov/exposurereport
The Centers for Disease Control and Prevention's *Third National Report on Human Exposure to Environmental Chemicals.*

www.greenerchoices.org/eco-labels/eco-good.cfm
Consumer Reports Greener Choices for products—covers everything from cars to food.

http://EnvironmentalChemistry.com/yogi/chemicals/
A chemical information database.

http://pesticideinfo.org
Pesticide Action Network's pesticide database.

http://hhs.gov
The U.S. Department of Health and Human Services' website provides information on health concerns and risks to the general public.

www.healthyhouseinstitute.com
"A resource for a better, safer indoor environment," this website includes information on everything from chemicals in personal-care and cleaning products to green living tips.

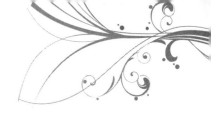

Appendix B:
Natural Ingredients List

Here is a closer look at some of the natural ingredients used in many of the products recommended in this book—and natural products in general—and their benefits for your skin and health:

almond*: See *sweet almond*

aloe vera (*Aloe barbadensis*) leaf extract/juice: Most commonly used to treat sunburn, aloe is an anti-inflammatory and increases collagen, which creates the youthful elasticity of skin. It is effective in toners and other face products as well. Aloe is one of the most soothing ingredients available and is applied to all types of burns, rashes, bites, and stings.

arrowroot (*Maranta arundinacea*) powder: Absorbs moisture and softens skin.

avocado (*Persea americana*) oil: A highly therapeutic oil that softens and moisturizes the skin, increases elasticity, and leaves no greasy residue. Avocado oil is primarily a monounsaturated oil. In contrast, polyunsaturated oils form greater amounts of free radicals, which are associated with rancidity. Although the oil is classed as a vegetable oil, the avocado is really a fruit, since it has a stone. It yields a rich and extremely deep-penetrating oil, filled with vitamins A, D, and E, lecithin, and potassium, known as the "youth mineral." It contains proteins, lecithin, beta-carotene, and more than 20 percent essential unsaturated fatty acids. The fatty acids contained in avocado oil are palmitic, palmitoleic, stearic, oleic, linoleic, and linolenic. It is also high in sterolins, which are reputed to reduce age spots and help heal sun damage and scars. The sterolins (also called plant steroids) in the oil help soften and moisturize the skin. It is an ideal ingredient for mature skin and for skin that is dehydrated, sun- or climate-damaged, as it assists in skin regeneration and rejuvenation and is easily absorbed into deep tissue. It also helps to relieve the dryness and itching of psoriasis and eczema.

algae (*Chlorophyta* sp.): Algae is high in amino acids, minerals, vitamins A, C, B-1, B-12, E, K, and D, and is used in skin care for its detoxifying, purifying, and hydrating effects. It is also said to regenerate cells and tissue.

apricot (*Prunus armeniaca*) oil: Apricot oil is a skin-softening oil that penetrates the skin easily without leaving a greasy, oily feeling. It is high in vitamins E and A, and rich in essential fatty acids. It is used to assist dry, irritated, mature, and sensitive skin.

beeswax (*Cera alba*): Beeswax is a natural wax that is used for many different applications. It can help emulsify, and it add firmness to oils when making balms and salves. It is also known for its ability to trap moisture in the skin; as an anti-bacterial, anti-microbial, and healing agent; and as a preservative.

borage seed oil (*Borago officinalis*): Borage oil has an extremely high content of essential fatty acids (EFAs), which are superior skin conditioners that help restore proper hydration to the skin. Borage oil is also the richest naturally occurring source of gamma linolenic acid (GLA), which is a fatty acid, and almost 20–26 percent of the oil is comprised of this fatty acid. It is used to help in reducing inflammation, the treatment of eczema, to moisturize itchy dry flaky skin, and to heal and reduce skin cuts and cracks.

bladder wrack (*Fucus vesiculosus*) extract: Bladder wrack is used for its antiviral, antibacterial, anti-inflammatory, and antioxidant benefits. It is a rich source of beta-carotene, potassium, and other minerals.

bilberry (*Vaccinium myrtillus*) extract: Bilberry extract contains vitamins A, B-1, B-2, C, and PP, and microelements that slow down skin aging. It has an antiinflammatory and soothing effect; its high vitamin content nourishes the skin. Its antioxidants reduce the action of free radicals and prevent damage of the phospholipid cell membrane.

black willow (*Salix nigra*) bark extract: This extract acts as a form of salicylic acid, a key ingredient in the treatment of acne, psoriasis, calluses, corns, keratosis, pilaris, and warts. It works by causing the cells of the epidermis to shed more readily, preventing pores from clogging and allowing room for new cell growth.

burdock (*Arctium lappa*) root extract: Burdock is an anti-inflammatory, antioxidant, and detoxifying agent.

calendula (*Calendula officinalis*) petals: Great for healing rashes, cuts, and wounds, calendula also reduces inflammation and removes excess oils from skin.

carrot (*Daucus carota*) seed oil: Carrot oil has superior skin benefits. It is filled with the highest concentration of carotenoids, over 550, making it an unsurpassed source of antioxidants. Carotenoids are antioxidants, delivered in a form that your skin can absorb and use. Antioxidants protect cells from free radicals that destroy healthy skin cells. Free radicals are caused by a many different factors. They can be the result of rancid oils stuck in your pores or environmental pollutants. If they are not eliminated, free radicals can damage cells, resulting in premature aging and a bevy of other skin issues.

chamomile (*Matricaria recutita*): Chamomile is widely used in skin care for its soothing, calming, and softening effects. It also contains flavonoids, which are an antioxidant.

chickweed (*Stellaria media*): A mild astringent, chickweed is used in many face products for its anti-inflammatory and soothing properties. It conditions skin and is used to treat psoriasis, eczema, rashes, and burns. Beyond face products, chickweed is also used on inflammatory conditions such as burns, stings, and itchy skin.

cocoa (*Theobroma cacao*) butter: One of the richest moisturizers on the market, cocoa butter can be applied in its pure form or used as a base for soaps, lotions, and creams. It is an especially appealing moisturizer because it melts at body temperature, so it can be stored in a bar but is still easily applied and absorbed into the skin. Cocoa butter creates a protective layer on the skin, which helps prevent environmental irritants. It is effective in treating dermatitis and eczema, as well as stretch marks. It has been used in the native countries of its origin for centuries, which speaks to its efficacy as a product.

coconut (*Cocos nucifera*) oil: An easily absorbed, nongreasy emollient, coconut oil boosts moisture in the skin so it is not easily evaporated. Coconut oil's antifungal properties make it ideal for moisturizing feet, but it is effective on the entire body. The benefits of coconut oil can be attributed to the presence of lauric acid and capric/caprylic acid, and it boasts antimicrobial, antioxidant, antifungal, antibacterial, and soothing properties.

deep-sea mud: This black mud frequently used in face masks is a homogenous mixture of Dead Sea mineral salts and organic elements (animal and vegetable) that form a kind of tarry clay. Applied to the skin, this clay stimulates and improves circulation. It also deeply cleanses and softens the skin. Its antimitotic and antiinflammatory properties are extremely useful in treating psoriasis.

eucalyptus (*Eucalyptus globulus*): Eucalyptus essential oil is used in bath, body, and skin care for its anti-inflammatory, healing, antiseptic, antibacterial, decongestant, and stimulating properties.

evening primrose (*Oenothera biennis*): This is an outstanding source of omega-6, an essential fatty acid (EFA). It is touted and used for rejuvenating skin, restoring hydration to severely dry skin, its antiaging properties, helping to repair skin damage at a cellular level, treating rosacea, and helping to maintain firmer skin.

French green clay: This clay consists of a variety of minerals and is usually formed by the weathering of rocks that contain silicone. Contrary to what its name suggests, French green clay comes from several places around the world and is one of the most common clays used in cosmetics. In a mask, clay acts as a sponge that soaks up excess oil so it can be washed away.

gingko (*Gingko biloba*): Gingko increases circulation, aids in the repair of collagen, and is filled with anti-oxidants, making it a widely used active ingredient in anti-aging skin-care products.

goat's milk: Goat's milk has long been recognized as a natural moisturizer and skin rejuvenator. In North America, when we hear the word *milk*, we instantly think of a dairy cow. In fact, worldwide, more people consume goat's milk than any other milk. From a nutritional standpoint, goat's milk and cow's milk are remarkably similar. However, there are significant differences in their proteins and fatty acids. The molecular structure of the proteins and fatty acids that predominate in cow's milk is much larger and longer than those in goat's milk, making them harder to digest. For those who are lactose-intolerant, goat's milk is frequently recommended as a substitute for cow's milk. Its protein structure also allows it to be easily absorbed and metabolized by your skin, making it the best milk for creating intense moisturizing and soothing results. Goat's milk is loaded with calcium, phosphorous, naturally occurring sodium, potassium, magnesium, vitamins A, B-1, B-2, B-3, and B-12, pantothenic acid, biotin, choline, and many other trace elements. When you use products made with goat's milk, you are nourishing not only your skin but also your entire body. Goat's milk is excellent for sensitive skin. People with eczema and psoriasis benefit from its nutrients.

grape (*Vitis vinifera*) seed oil: Grape seed oil is a preferred cosmetic ingredient for damaged and stressed tissues, possessing regenerative and restructuring qualities that enhance moisturizing. It can help skin retain the normal structure of epithelium cells and nerve cells by supporting the cell membranes, as well as restoring collagen. It is noted to be especially effective for repair of the skin around the eyes. Used as an all-over moisturizer, grape seed oil is known to minimize stretch marks. A light, thin oil, it leaves a glossy film over the skin when used as a carrier for essential oils in aromatherapy. It also contains more linoleic acid—an omega-6 fatty acid that contains both tocopherol and retinol, antioxidants that prevent signs of aging and can restore and heal damaged skin—than many other carrier oils.

green tea (*Camellia sinensis*): Vitamins C and E make green tea a powerful antioxidant. Green tea also has anti-inflammatory and antiaging properties. Green tea destroys free radicals and helps protect skin from damaging environmental exposure.

guar gum: A thickener extracted from the seeds of the guar shrub, guar gum is a naturally occurring alternative to human-made (but harmless) xanthan gum.

jojoba (*Simmondsia chinensis*) nut oil: Jojoba oil is actually a wax that mimics the natural sebum (oil) our body produces. It is also easily absorbed and does not clog pores. For people with oily skin, jojoba helps balance and restore the skin's own natural oil production. Applying small amounts of jojoba actually decreases oil production in overactive skin. It softens skin, reduces wrinkles, and helps promote the growth of new skin cells.

lemon (*Citrus medica limonum*): Lemons have astringent properties, tightening pores to keep dirt and oils out and give skin a smooth, healthy glow.

lichen (*Usnea barbata*) extract: Lichen is an antibiotic, antibacterial, and antimicrobial agent.

licorice (*Glykyrrhiza glabra*) root: Licorice root is an anti-inflammatory, antifungal, antibacterial, antiviral, and antioxidant agent.

mango (*Mangifera indica*) butter: Like cocoa butter, mango butter melts on contact with skin. In addition to this obvious perk, mango butter has many beneficial qualities. It is used in the tropics for moisturizing and protecting the skin, as well as for soothing bites and stings. It is effective in relieving itching and damaged skin, and it can help treat the symptoms of sunburns, dermatitis, and eczema, as well as reduce stretch marks.

neem (*Melia azadirachta*) seed oil: Neem seed oil has been used for centuries in Bangladeshi medicine to assist in the healing of topical skin disorders such as eczema, psoriasis, rashes, acne, burns, and tinea. It is rich in fatty acids and glycerides, and it provides an excellent natural moisturizing base for skin-care formulations.

nettle (*Urtica dioica*) leaf: Nettles are an anti-inflammatory, as well as a valuable source of beta-carotene; vitamins A, C and E; iron; calcium; phosphates; minerals; and amino acids.

oats (*Avena sativa*): Oats are used for the treatment of many different skin problems and disorders, such as redness and swelling, acne, eczema, and psoriasis. They can be used in creams, lotions, bath preparations, and cleansers. In creams and lotions, they help restore moisture and calm redness. With benefits ranging from soothing to moisturizing, oats can be used in everything from bath soaks for both eczema and psoriasis to masks, lotions, and hair care.

olive (*Olea europaea*) leaf extract or oil: Olive leaf extracts boast antimicrobial and antiaging properties. They are often used in products for their ability to heal damaged or wounded skin. Olive increases blood flow and stimulates skin-cell regeneration.

orange (*Citrus aurantium dulcis* or *Citrus sinensis*): Oranges have astringent properties, tightening pores to keep dirt and oils out and give skin a smooth, healthy glow.

papaya (*Carica papaya*) extract: Papaya is rich in both antioxidants (vitamins A and C) and enzymes. Its potent fruit enzymes gently exfoliate your skin by "digesting" the dead skin cells.

pistachio (*Pistacia vera*) oil*: Thanks to its high vitamin content, pistachio oil nourishes, softens, and hydrates the skin. Since it is easily absorbed by the skin, it is often used in massage.

plantain (*Plantago* sp.) fruit: High in magnesium, potassium, iron, zinc, and vitamins A, B, E, and F, plantain is a rich source of nutrients for your skin. It also softens, soothes, and calms skin that is red or irritated.

potassium sorbate: A naturally occurring, food-grade preservative, used for maintaining the potency and active properties of ingredients.

pumpkin (*Cucurbita pepo*): Beneficial for all skin types, especially environmentally damaged or sensitive skin, pumpkin is high in vitamin A (skin healing), vitamin C (antioxidant), and zinc. It soothes, moisturizes, and acts as a carrier, assisting absorption and intensifying the results of the product.

rooibos (*Aspalathus linearis*) leaves: Used to treat acne, rooibos is also highly beneficial for skin in general. It contains minerals, flavonoids, thirty-seven natural antioxidants, vitamin C, and alpha hydroxy acids.

rose-hip (*Rosa canina*) seed oil/extract: Rose-hip oil contains natural tretinoin, a derivative of vitamin A, and is proven to delay the effects of skin aging. It aids in cell regeneration and boosts collagen levels to make skin smoother and firmer. It is also high in vitamin C, and all of its natural vitamins exist in a form that your skin can actually use and receive benefits from.

rose (*Rosa canina*) water: Good for all skin types, rose water is especially valuable for dry, sensitive, or aging skin. It has a tonic and astringent effect on the capillaries just below the skin surface, which makes it useful in diminishing the redness caused by enlarged capillaries. It is also soothing to the nerves and is regarded as a mild sedative and antidepressant.

rosemary (*Rosmarinus officinalis*) leaf extract or oil: Applied to the skin, rosemary essential oil helps strengthen the capillaries and has a rejuvenating effect. Often used for its antiseptic, antimicrobial, and antioxidant properties, rosemary is also a powerful astringent, tightening pores and preventing dirt and oils from entering.

seaweed (*Fucus sp.*): Seaweed stimulates circulation; revitalizes, hydrates, nourishes, and detoxifies skin; and firms the skin. It is filled with skin-loving ingredients such as amino acids, vitamins, lipids, proteins, and minerals. These ingredients exist in seaweed in a form that is easily absorbed and used by your skin.

shiitake mushroom (*Lentinula edodes*): Shiitake mushrooms contain the antioxidant L-ergothioneine, which helps prevent cell breakdown and exfoliate the skin. They are used to reduce inflammation and to prevent the appearance of fine lines and wrinkles. They also boost collagen production and are high in kojic acid, a natural skin lightener.

sesame (*Sesamum indicum*) oil: Sesame oil is naturally high in vitamins A and E, proteins, and linoleic acid (an essential fatty acid).

shea (*Butyrospermum parkii*) butter: Made from the nuts of the karite, or shea, tree, which is native to Central and West Africa, shea is a thick butter filled with fatty acids that penetrates the skin and is wonderful for healing cracked or flaky skin. It also helps heal burns, sores, scars, dermatitis, psoriasis, and dandruff, reduces stretch marks, promotes cell renewal, increases circulation, and protects the skin from ultraviolet rays and environmental and free-radical damage. Shea butter is used in the production of many creams, lotions, soaps, and shampoos.

sodium benzoate: A food-grade preservative, sodium benzoate is recognized as safe for consumption and is used for maintaining the potency and active properties of other ingredients.

stearic acid: A fatty acid used to thicken products. While it is a harmless, food-grade substance that can easily be derived from a vegetable source, it is sometimes unnecessarily derived from animal products, so try to determine the source used in your products.

sweet almond (*Prunus amygdalus dulcis*) oil*: Almond oil makes creams and lotions smooth and easy to spread and leaves skin silky and soft. Due to its emollient properties, this oil is suitable for all skin types but is especially good for dry skin because it helps relieve itching and irritation. This expeller-pressed oil contains vitamins A, B-1, B-2, B-6, and E, and is considered nonirritating. It acts as an excellent base oil for many products.

tamanu*: Tamanu heals scarring and is used to treat cuts, burns, acne, bites, stretch marks, psoriasis, athlete's foot, infected nails, diaper rash, age spots, arthritis, joint pain, blisters, wounds and sores, rashes, herpes, ringworm, chapped lips, and cracked, dry skin. It works as a moisturizer, antibiotic, antiinflammatory, and antifungal, as well as promoting tissue healing.

vegetable glycerin: Vegetable glycerin has emollient properties, which soften and soothe the skin, and assist the outer epidermis in retaining moisture.

vitamin A: Vitamin A is an effective treatment for acne. Its antioxidant properties help protect skin from environmental irritants and free radicals. It regulates oil, so while it helps reduce oil in oily skin, it does not remove moisture from dry skin. It keeps pores open and clean and has slight antibacterial properties. It helps heal and repair skin.

vitamin C: Vitamin C is an antioxidant and helps prevent the oils in your skin from going rancid. Rancid oils break down collagen and accelerate aging. Vitamin C can also boost the production of collagen, an essential protein that keeps skin firm and toned. When collagen is not produced properly, skin can begin to sag and lose its vitality. Collagen is also an important element in the health of the connective tissue throughout your body. Bringing this nutrient into your diet and skin-care plan can help you look and feel better, reduce wrinkles, and improve your skin's overall quality.

vitamin E: Vitamin E is vital in protecting skin cells from ultraviolet light, pollution, drugs, and other elements that produce cell-damaging free radicals. It helps skin look younger by reducing the appearance of fine lines and wrinkles. It is used to treat acne, and studies have shown that it might help skin recover from acne scarring. Vitamin E regulates our levels of retinol, or vitamin A, which is essential for healthy skin. Decreases in retinol levels cause the oxidation of unsaturated fatty acids in the cells, which causes toxic effects. Vitamin E curbs this oxidation process and restores normal levels of retinol.

wheat (*Triticum vulgare*) germ oil: Rich in vitamins A, E, and D and essential fatty acids, wheat germ oil also contains squalene, a natural antibacterial involved in cell growth that boasts great healing properties. Wheat germ oil is applied topically to promote the formation of new cells and improve circulation, and it is said to help repair sun damage. It is also used to help relieve the symptoms of dermatitis, and its nourishing properties are most useful in treating dry, sensitive skin. There are different opinions about whether people with celiac disease should avoid wheat germ oil; I would, just to be safe.

witch hazel (*Hamamelis virginiana*) extract/distillate: Very different from the witch hazel that you buy in the store, which is between 50 and 85 percent alcohol, true witch hazel (witch hazel distillate) is fantastic for your skin. It has very strong astringent and tonic properties and reduces redness, rashes, itching, swelling, and scaling. In addition, it heals cracked or blistered skin and soothes the symptoms of eczema and psoriasis. It is a powerful anti-inflammatory and an effective wound wash and antiseptic; it can be used to soothe bites and stings. It is also coveted for its antiaging properties.

* If you have nut allergies, consult with you doctor before using any nut products, such as tamanu, pistachio, and almond.

Appendix C:
Toxic Ingredients List

Source: Adapted from "Toxic Chemical Ingredient Detective" (http://www .health-report.co.uk/ingredients-directory.htm). Please note this material is from a British article, and our MSDSs in the United States may differ slightly.

In terms of your safety as a consumer, the material in this Appendix and the list of "The Top Ten Ingredients to Avoid" on page 32 are possibly the most important pieces of information for you to refer to. For a downloadable copy of the list and this Appendix go to www.hunterhouse.com.

1,4-dioxane: A carcinogenic contaminant of cosmetic products. Almost 50 percent of cosmetics containing ethoxylated surfactants were found to contain dioxane. See *ethoxylated surfactants.*

From the material safety data sheet (MSDS):

1,4-dioxane may exert its effects through inhalation, skin absorption, and ingestion.

1,4-dioxane is listed as a carcinogen.

Effects of overexposure: 1,4-dioxane is an eye and mucous membrane irritant, primary skin irritant, central nervous system depressant, nephrotoxin, and hepatotoxin.

Acute exposure causes irritation, headache, dizziness, and narcosis. Chronic inhalation exposure can produce damage to the liver and kidneys, and blood disorders.

Medical condition aggravated by exposure: preclude from exposure those individuals with disease of the blood, liver, kidneys, central nervous system, and susceptible to dermatitis.

2-bromo-2-nitropropane-1,3-diol (bronopol): Toxic, causes allergic contact dermatitis.

alcohol, isopropyl (SD-40): A very drying and irritating solvent and dehydrator that strips the skin's natural acid mantle, making us more vulnerable to bacteria, molds, and viruses. It is made from propylene, a petroleum derivative. It may promote brown spots and premature aging of skin.

ammonium laureth sulfate (ALES): See *anionic surfactants.* See *sodium laureth sulfate.* See *nitrosating agents.*

ammonium lauryl sulfate (ALS): See *anionic surfactants.* See *sodium laureth sulfate.* See *nitrosating agents.*

anionic surfactants: *Anionic* refers to the negative charge these surfactants have. They may be contaminated with nitrosamines, which are carcinogenic. Surfactants can pose serious health threats. They are used in car washes, as garage-floor cleaners, and as engine degreasers—and in 90 percent of personal-care products that foam. The following are examples of anionic surfactants:

- sodium lauryl sulfate (SLS)
- sodium laureth sulfate (SLES)
- ammonium lauryl sulfate (ALS)
- ammonium laureth sulfate (ALES)
- sodium methyl cocoyl taurate
- sodium lauryl sarcosinate
- sodium cocoyl sarcosinate
- potassium coco hydrolyzed collagen
- TEA (triethanolamine) lauryl sulfate
- TEA (triethanolamine) laureth sulfate
- lauryl or cocoyl sarcosine
- disodium oleamide sulfosuccinate
- disodium laureth sulfosuccinate
- disodium dioctyl sulfosuccinate

benzalkonium chloride: Highly toxic, primary skin irritant. See *cationic surfactants.*

From the material safety data sheet (MSDS):

Material is highly toxic via oral route.

Effects of overexposure: Mists can cause irritation to the skin, eyes, nose, throat, and mucous membranes. Avoid direct contact. Symptoms: Muscular paralysis, low blood pressure, central nervous system depression, and weakness.

Emergency and first aid procedures:

Eyes: Corrosive! Immediately wash eyes with plenty of water.

Inhalation: Remove person to fresh air. Give oxygen (if breathing is difficult). Call physician.

Ingestion: If conscious, immediately drink large quantities of fluid to dilute and induce vomiting. Call physician.

butylated hydroxyanisole (BHA): Dr. Epstein reports in his book *Unreasonable Risk* that this chemical is carcinogenic. It is also known to cause allergic contact dermatitis.

butylated hydroxytoluene (BHT): Causes allergic contact dermatitis. It contains toluene.

cationic surfactants: These chemicals have a positive electrical charge. They contain a quaternary ammonium group and are often called "quats." These are used in hair conditioners, but they originated in the paper and fabric industries as softeners and antistatic agents. In the long run, they cause the hair to become dry and brittle. They are synthetic, irritating, allergenic, and toxic, and oral intake of them can be lethal.

- stearalkonium chloride
- benzalkonium chloride
- cetrimonium chloride
- cetalkonium chloride
- lauryl dimonium hydrolyzed collagen

cetalkonium chloride: See *cationic surfactants.*

cetrimonium chloride: See *cationic surfactants.*

chloromethylisothiazolinone: Causes contact dermatitis.

cocoamidopropyl betaine: From the material safety data sheet (MSDS): "Can cause eye and skin irritation."

cocoyl sarcosine: See *nitrosating agents.*

cyclomethicone: See *silicone-derived emollients.*

DEA (diethanolamine), MEA (monoethanolamine), and **TEA (triethanolamine):** Often used in cosmetics to adjust the pH, and used with many fatty acids to convert acid to salt (stearate), which then becomes the base for a cleanser. TEA causes allergic reactions, including eye problems, dryness of hair and skin, and could be toxic if absorbed into the body over a long period of time.

These chemicals are already restricted in Europe due to known carcinogenic effects. Dr. Samuel Epstein (Professor of Environmental Health at the University of Illinois) says that "Repeated skin applications...of DEA-based detergents resulted in a major increase in the incidence of liver and kidney cancer." *See* nitrosating agents.

From the material safety data sheet (MSDS):

Health Hazard Acute and Chronic: "Product is severely irritating to body tissues and possibly corrosive to the eyes."

Explanation Carcinogenicity: Amines react with nitrosating agents to form nitrosamines, which are carcinogenic.

diazolidinyl urea: Established as a primary cause of contact dermatitis (American Academy of Dermatology). This contains formaldehyde, a carcinogenic chemical, is toxic by inhalation, a strong irritant, and causes contact dermatitis. See *formaldehyde*.

From the material safety data sheet (MSDS):

Causes severe eye irritation. May cause skin irritation. Signs and symptoms of exposure:

Symptoms of inhalation: If misted, will cause irritation of mucous membranes, nose, eyes, and throat. Coughing, difficulty in breathing.

Symptoms of skin contact: Contact causes smarting and burning sensations, inflammation, burns, painful blisters. Profound damage to tissue.

Symptoms of eye contact: Will cause painful burning or stinging of eyes and lids, watering of eyes, and inflammation of conjunctiva.

dimethicone: See *silicone-derived emollients*.

dimethicone copolyol: See *silicone-derived emollients*.

disodium dioctyl sulfosuccinate: See *anionic surfactants*.

disodium laureth sulfosuccinate: See *anionic surfactants*. See *ethoxylated surfactants*.

disodium oleamide sulfosuccinate: See *anionic surfactants*.

DMDM hydantoin: Contains formaldehyde. See *formaldehyde*.

ethoxylated surfactants: Ethoxylated surfactants are widely used in cosmetics as foaming agents, emulsifiers and humectants. As part of the manufacturing process, the toxic chemical 1,4-dioxane, a potent carcinogen, is generated.

On the label, they are identified by the prefix "PEG," "polyethylene," "polyethylene glycol," "polyoxyethylene," "-eth-," or "-oxynol-." See *1, 4-dioxane*.

FD&C Color Pigments: Synthetic colors made from coal tar. These contain heavy metal salts that deposit toxins onto the skin, causing skin sensitivity and irritation. Animal studies have shown almost all of them to be carcinogenic.

formaldehyde: Formaldehyde is a known carcinogen (causes cancer). It causes allergic, irritant and contact dermatitis, headaches, and chronic fatigue. The vapor is extremely irritating to the eyes, nose, and throat (mucous membranes). See *nitrosating agents.*

fragrance: *Fragrance* on a label can indicate the presence of up to four thousand separate ingredients, many toxic or carcinogenic. Symptoms reported to the U.S. FDA include headaches, dizziness, allergic rashes, skin discoloration, violent coughing and vomiting, and skin irritation. Clinical observation proves fragrances can affect the central nervous system, causing depression, hyperactivity, and irritability.

hydrolyzed animal protein: See *nitrosating agents.*

imidazolidinyl urea: The trade name for this chemical is Germall 155. It releases formaldehyde, a carcinogenic chemical, into cosmetics over 10°C. See *formaldehyde.* See *nitrosating agents.*

isopropyl palmitate [isopropylpalmitate]: A fatty acid from palm oil combined with synthetic alcohol. Industry tests on rabbits indicate the chemical can cause skin irritation and dermatitis. Also shown to be comedogenic (acne-promoting).

isothiazolinone: Causes contact dermatitis.
From the material safety data sheet (MSDS):

Eye contact: Corrosive to the eyes with possible permanent damage.

Skin contact: Corrosive to the skin, possibly resulting in third-degree burns. Can be harmful if absorbed. Can cause allergic contact dermatitis in susceptible individuals.

Ingestion: can be fatal.

Inhalation: Can be corrosive to the mucous membranes and the lungs. Can cause an allergic reaction in susceptible individuals.

lanolin: Any chemicals used on sheep will contaminate the lanolin obtained from the wool. The majority of lanolin used in cosmetics is highly contaminated with organo-phosphate pesticides and insecticides.

lauryl dimonium hydrolyzed collagen: See *cationic surfactants.*

lauryl or cocoyl sarcosine: See *anionic surfactants.*

lauryl sarcosine: See *nitrosating agents.*

liquidum paraffinum: Liquidum paraffinum is an exotic-sounding way to say mineral oil. See *mineral oil.*

MEA compounds: See *nitrosating agents.*

methylisothiazolinone and methylchloroisothiazolinone: Both cause cosmetic allergies and potential dangerous neuro-toxic effects.

According to senior author Elias Aizenman, professor of neurobiology at the University of Pittsburgh School of Medicine:

> "While more research is needed to determine what effect MIT would have in rodent models, both at the cellular level and to a developing nervous system, our results thus far suggest there is potential that everyday exposure to the chemical could also be harmful to humans. I would be particularly concerned about occupational exposure in pregnant women and the possibility of risk to the fetus.

> "As an antimicrobial agent, or biocide, MIT and related compounds kill harmful bacteria that like to grow near moisture or water and hence, often are found in personal-care products, as well as in water-cooling systems; however, the research has now revealed that even a 10-minute exposure at a high concentration was lethal to the nerve cells.

> "This chemical is being used more and more extensively, yet there have been no neurotoxicity studies in humans to indicate what kind and at what level exposure is safe. I realize it's a big leap to suggest there may be a parallel between environmental exposure and the noticeably higher rates of diagnosed childhood developmental disabilities, but I would caution, that based on our data, there very well could be neuro-developmental consequences from MIT. Clearly, more study is needed, with both scientists and government regulators equally engaged."

mineral oil: Petroleum by-product that coats the skin like a plastic, clogging the pores. This ingredient interferes with skin's ability to eliminate toxins and promotes acne and other disorders. It slows down skin function and cell development, resulting in premature aging. It is used in many products (baby oil is 100 percent mineral oil!). Any mineral oil derivative can be contaminated with cancer-causing PAHs (polycyclic aromatic hydrocarbons). Manufacturers use petrolatum because it is unbelievably cheap.

- mineral oil
- paraffin wax
- liquidum paraffinum (also known as posh mineral oil)
- paraffin oil
- petrolatum

nitrosating agents: The following chemicals can cause nitrosamine contamination, which have been determined to form cancer in laboratory animals. There are wide and repeated concerns in the United States and Europe about the contamination of cosmetics products with nitrosamines.

- cocoyl sarcosine
- imidazolidinyl urea
- hydrolyzed animal protein
- MEA compounds
- sodium lauryl sulfate
- sodium laureth sulfate
- sodium methyl cocoyl taurate
- 2-bromo-2-nitropropane-1,3-diol

- DEA compounds
- formaldehyde
- lauryl sarcosine
- quaternium-7, 15, 31, 60, etc.
- ammonium lauryl sulfate
- ammonium laureth sulfate
- TEA compounds

paraben preservatives (methyl-, propyl-, butyl-, and ethyl-): Used as inhibitors of microbial growth and to extend the shelf life of products. These are widely used even though they are known to be toxic. They have caused many allergic reactions and skin rashes. This ingredient is highly toxic.

From the material safety data sheet (MSDS):

Emergency overview:

Warning! Harmful if swallowed or inhaled. Causes irritation to skin, eyes and respiratory tract. May cause allergic skin reaction.

Skin contact: Causes irritation to skin. Symptoms include redness, itching, and pain. May cause allergic skin reactions.

Eye contact: Causes irritation, redness, and pain.

paraffin wax/oil: Paraffin wax is mineral oil wax. See *mineral oil.*

phthalates: Toxic chemicals used as a plasticizers in food wraps and many pliable plastics and containers. They are also used in hair sprays and some cosmetics, including nail varnishes—areas from which they are readily absorbed into the system. All 289 people in a recent test for body load of chemicals tested positive for phthalates. Phthalates are implicated with low sperm counts and also for causing sexual abnormalities and deformities.

polyethylene glycol (PEG) compounds: Potentially carcinogenic petroleum ingredients that can alter and reduce the skin's natural moisture factor. This could increase the appearance of aging and leave you more vulnerable to bacteria. This ingredient is used in cleansers to dissolve oil and grease. These ingredients adjust the melting point and thicken products. They are also used in caustic spray-on oven cleaners. See *ethoxylated surfactants.*

potassium coco hydrolyzed collagen: See *anionic surfactants.*

propylene/butylene glycol: Propylene glycol (PG) is a petroleum derivative. It penetrates the skin and can weaken protein and cellular structure. It is commonly used to make extracts from herbs. PG is strong enough to remove barnacles from boats! The EPA considers PG so toxic that it requires workers to wear protective gloves, clothing, and goggles and to dispose of any PG solutions by burying them in the ground. Because PG penetrates the skin so quickly, the EPA warns against skin contact to prevent consequences such as brain, liver, and kidney abnormalities. But there isn't even a warning label on products, such as stick deodorants, where the concentration is greater than in most industrial products.

From the material safety data sheet (MSDS):

Health Hazard Acute and Chronic

Inhalation: May cause respiratory and throat irritation, central nervous system depression, blood and kidney disorders. May cause nystagmus, lymphocytosis.

Skin: Irritation and dermatitis, absorption.

Eyes: Irritation and conjunctivitis.

Ingestion: Pulmonary edema, brain damage, hypoglycemia, intravascular hemolysis. Death may occur.

PVP/VA copolymer: A petroleum-derived chemical used in hair sprays, wave sets, and other cosmetics. It can be considered toxic, since particles may contribute to foreign bodies in the lungs of sensitive persons.

quaternium-7, -15, -31, -60, etc.: Toxic, cause skin rashes and allergic reactions. Formaldehyde releasers. Dr. Epstein reports in his book *Unreasonable Risk*, "Substantive evidence of casual relation to leukemia, multiple myeloma, non-Hodgkin's lymphoma, and other cancers." See *nitrosating agents*.

From the material safety data sheet (MSDS):

Skin: Prolonged or repeated exposure may cause skin irritation. May cause more severe response if skin is damp.

May be a weak skin sensitizer in susceptible individuals at greater than 1 percent in aqueous solution.

rancid natural emollients: Natural oils used in cosmetics should be cold pressed. The refined vegetable oils found on supermarket shelves and many health food stores which lack color, odor, and taste are devoid of nutrients, essential fatty acids, vitamins, and unsaponifiables—all valuable skin-conditioning agents! They also contain poisonous "trans" fatty acids as a result of the refining process.

Another important factor to consider with creams made from plant oil is the use-by date. The most beneficial plant oils (like rose-hip, borage, and evening primrose oils) are polyunsaturated, which means they oxidize and go rancid fairly quickly (about six months). Most off-the-shelf cosmetics have a shelf life of three years. Rancid oils are harmful, and they form free radicals, which damage and age your skin.

silicone-derived emollients: Silicone emollients are occlusive—that is, they coat the skin, trapping anything beneath it, and they do not allow the skin to breathe (much like plastic wrap would do).

Recent studies have indicated that prolonged exposure of the skin to sweat, by occlusion, causes skin irritation. Some synthetic emollients are known tumor promoters and accumulate in the liver and lymph nodes. They are also nonbiodegradable, causing negative environmental impact.

- dimethicone
- dimethicone copolyol
- cyclomethicone

Silicone was and still is used in breast implants. Tens of thousands of women with breast implants have complained of debilitating symptoms. Anecdotal evidence indicates silicone to be toxic to the human body.

sodium cocoyl sarcosinate: See *anionic surfactants*.

sodium hydroxide: Also known as caustic soda. A powerful alkali used in industry for cleaning drains and pipe lines, also used in oven cleaners. Workers exposed to steam containing sodium hydroxide have suffered lung damage and an increased risk of throat cancer. This ingredient is used in toothpastes and as a pH adjuster in skin creams. It causes contact dermatitis and may sensitize individuals to other chemicals.

From the material safety data sheet (MSDS):

Poison! Danger! Corrosive. May be fatal if swallowed. Harmful if inhaled. Causes burns to any area of contact. Reacts with water, acids, and other materials.

Ingestion: Corrosive! Swallowing may cause severe burns of mouth, throat, and stomach. Severe scarring of tissue and death may result. Symptoms may include bleeding, vomiting, diarrhea, and a fall in blood pressure. Damage may appear days after exposure.

Skin contact: Corrosive! Contact with skin can cause irritation or severe burns and scarring with greater exposures.

Eye contact: Corrosive! Causes irritation of eyes, and with greater exposures it can cause burns that may result in permanent impairment of vision, even blindness.

Chronic exposure: Prolonged contact with diluted solutions has a destructive effect upon tissue.

Aggravation of preexisting conditions: Persons with preexisting skin disorders or eye problems or impaired respiratory function may be more susceptible to the effects of the substance.

sodium laureth sulfate (SLES): When combined with other chemicals, SLES and ammonium laureth sulfate (ALES) can create nitrosamines, a potent class of carcinogens. It is frequently disguised in seminatural cosmetics with the explanation "comes from coconut."

See *anionic surfactants.* See *ethoxylated surfactants.* See *nitrosating agents.*

From the material safety data sheet (MSDS):

"Warning! Causes skin and eye irritation! Avoid contact with eyes, skin, and clothing. The material was classified as a moderate-to-severe eye irritant."

sodium lauryl sarcosinate: See *anionic surfactants.*

sodium lauryl sulfate (SLS): Used in car washes, garage floor cleaners, and engine degreasers—and in 90 percent of products that foam.

Animals exposed to SLS and ammonium lauryl sulfate (ALS) experience eye damage, central nervous system depression, labored breathing, diarrhea, severe skin irritation, and even death.

Young eyes may not develop properly if exposed to SLS and ALS, because proteins are dissolved. SLS and ALS may also damage the skin's immune system by causing layers to separate and inflame. It is frequently disguised in seminatural cosmetics with the explanation "comes from coconut." See *nitrosating agents.* See *anionic surfactants.*

From the material safety data sheet (MSDS):

"Severe skin irritant."

sodium methyl cocoyl taurate: See *nitrosating agents.* See *anionic surfactants.*

stearalkonium chloride: A chemical used in hair conditioners and creams. Causes allergic reactions. Stearalkonium chloride was developed by the fabric industry as a fabric softener, and it is a lot cheaper and easier to use in hair-conditioning formulas than proteins or herbals that do help hair health. Toxic. See *cationic surfactants.*

talc: Scientific studies have shown that routine application of talcum powder in the genital area is associated with a three-to-fourfold increase in the development of ovarian cancer.

TEA (triethanolamine) laureth sulfate: Synthetic emulsifier. Highly acidic. Over 40 percent of cosmetics containing triethanolamine (TEA) have been found to be contaminated with nitrosamines, which are potent carcinogens.

From material safety data sheet (MSDS):

Special hazard precautions: Product is severely irritating to body tissues and possibly corrosive to the eyes. Handle with care. Avoid eye and skin contact. Avoid breathing vapors if generated. If there is danger of eye contact, wear a face shield.

Explanation carcinogenicity: Amines react with nitrosating agents to form nitrosoamines, which are carcinogenic.

See *anionic surfactants*. See *nitrosating agents*.

TEA compounds: See *nitrosating agents*.

toluene: From the material safety data sheet (MSDS):

Poison! Danger! Harmful or fatal if swallowed. Harmful if inhaled or absorbed through skin. Vapor harmful. Flammable liquid and vapor. May affect liver, kidneys, blood system, or central nervous system. Causes irritation to skin, eyes, and respiratory tract.

Inhalation: Inhalation may cause irritation of the upper respiratory tract. Symptoms of overexposure may include fatigue, confusion, headache, dizziness and drowsiness. Peculiar skin sensations (e.g., pins and needles) or numbness may be produced. Very high concentrations may cause unconsciousness and death.

Ingestion: Swallowing may cause abdominal spasms and other symptoms that parallel overexposure from inhalation. Aspiration of material into the lungs can cause chemical pneumonitis, which may be fatal.

Skin contact: Causes irritation. May be absorbed through skin.

Eye contact: Causes severe eye irritation with redness and pain.

Chronic exposure: reports of chronic poisoning describe anemia, decreased blood cell count, and bone marrow hypoplasia. Liver and kidney damage may occur. Repeated or prolonged contact has a defatting action, causing drying, redness, and dermatitis.

Exposure to toluene may affect the developing fetus.

triethanolamine: From the material safety data sheet:

May cause eye irritation.

Skin contact: Prolonged exposure not likely to cause significant eye irritation. Repeated exposure may cause irritation, even a burn.

Eye contact: May cause moderate eye irritation. Corneal injury is unlikely.

Skin sensitization: Skin contact may cause an allergic skin reaction in a small proportion of individuals.

Effects of repeated exposure: In animals, effects have been reported on the following organs: kidney; liver.

Bibliography

Books and Journal Articles

Angeloglou, Maggie. *A History of Make-up.* New York: Macmillan, 1970.

Babich, Michael A. "The Risk of Chronic Toxicity Associated with Exposure to Diisononyl Phthalate (DINP) in Children's Products." U.S. Consumer Product Safety Commission. December 1998. *Epidemiology and Health Sciences.* http://www.cpsc.gov/phth/risk.pdf www.cpsc.gov/phth/risk.pdf] (accessed 15 August 2008).

Blood, D. C., and V. P. Studdert, and C. C. Gay. *Saunders Comprehensive Veterinary Dictionary*, 3rd Ed. Philadelphia, PA: Saunders Ltd., 2006. http://medical-dictionary.thefreedictionary.com (accessed 25 August 2008).

Brand, Peg Zeglin. *Beauty Matters.* Bloomington: Indiana University Press, 2000.

Callaghan, Karen A. *Ideals of Feminine Beauty: Philosophical, Social, and Cultural.* Westport, CT: Greenwood Press, 1994.

Centers for Disease Control and Prevention. "Spotlight on Phthalates." Atlanta: Centers for Disease Control, 2005. NCEH Pub 05-0664. http://www.cdc.gov/ExposureReport/pdf/factsheet_phthalates.pdf.

Centers for Disease Control and Prevention. *Third National Report on Human Exposure to Environmental Chemicals.* Atlanta: Centers for Disease Control, 2005. http://www.cdc.gov/exposurereport (accessed 26 July 2008).

Center for Food Safety and Applied Nutrition, Office of Cosmetics and Colors. "Phthalates and Cosmetic Products." Washington, DC: Center for Food Safety and Applied Nutrition, Office of Cosmetics and Colors, 19 April 2001. http://www.cfsan.fda.gov/%7Edms/cos-phth.html (accessed 1 June 2009).

Center for Food Safety and Applied Nutrition, Office of Cosmetics and Colors. "FDA Authority Over Cosmetics." Washington, DC: Center for

Food Safety and Applied Nutrition, Office of Cosmetics and Colors, 3 March 2005. http://www.cfsan.fda.gov/~dms/cos-206.html

Cobb, Vicky. *The Secret Life of Cosmetics: A Science Experiment Book*. New York: Lippincott, 1985.

Corson, Richard. *Fashions in Makeup: From Ancient to Modern Times*. New York: Universe Books, 1972.

Curry, Walter Clyde. *The Middle English Ideal of Personal Beauty: As Found in the Metrical Romances, Chronicles, and Legends of the XIII, XIV, and XV Centuries*. Baltimore: J. H. Furst, 1916.

Dawson, Mildred Leinweber. *Beauty Lab: How Science Is Changing the Way We Look*. New York: Silver Moon Press, 1996.

DiGangi, Joseph, et al. "Aggregate Exposure to Phthalates in Humans." Health Care Without Harm. July 2002. http://www.noharm.org/library/docs/Phthalate_Report.pdf www.noharm.org/library/docs/Phthalate_Report.pdf] (accessed August 2008).

Environmental Working Group. "Body Burden: The Pollution in Newborns." Washington, DC: Environmental Working Group, July 2005. http://www.ewg.org/reports/bodyburden2 (accessed 1 June 2009).

Epstein, Samuel S., and Richard D. Grundy. *Consumer Health and Product Hazards: Cosmetics and Drugs, Pesticides, Food Additives*. Cambridge: MIT Press, 1974.

Harrison, Roy M., and R. E. Hester. *Endocrine Disrupting Chemicals*. Cambridge, U.K.: Royal Society of Chemistry, 1999.

Hogarth, William. *The Analysis of Beauty*. London: Scolar Press, 1974.

Howard, Phillip H. *Handbook of Environmental Fate and Exposure Data for Organic Chemicals*. Chelsea, MI: Lewis Publishers, 1989.

Kenneth Barbalace. Chemical Database: http://environmentalchemistry.com. 1995–2008. (Accessed 25 August 2008).

Kovach, Francis J. *Philosophy of Beauty*. Norman: University of Oklahoma Press, 1974.

Leung, Albert Y. *Encyclopedia of Common Natural Ingredients Used in Food, Drugs, and Cosmetics*. 2d ed. New York: John Wiley & Sons, 1996.

Lewis, Grace Ross. *1001 Chemicals in Everyday Products*. New York: Wiley, 1999.

Lewis, Richard J., Sr. *Hazardous Chemicals Desk Reference.* 4th ed. New York, Van Nostrand Reinhold, 1997.

Nater, Johan P., and Dhiam H. Liem. *Unwanted Effects of Cosmetics and Drugs Used in Dermatology.* New York: Elsevier, 1985.

Palma, Robert J., Sr., and Mark Espenscheid. *The Complete Guide to Household Chemicals.* Amherst, NY: Prometheus Books, 1995.

Peiss, Kathy Lee. *Hope in a Jar: The Making of America's Beauty Culture.* New York: Metropolitan Books, 1998.

Robson, Mark, and William Toscano. *Risk Assessment for Environmental Health.* San Francisco: Jossey-Bass, 2007.

Rose, Jeanne. *Kitchen Cosmetics: Using Herbs, Fruits, and Eatables in Natural Cosmetics.* San Francisco: Panjandrum/Aris Books, 1978.

Scranton, Philip. *Beauty and Business: Commerce, Gender, and Culture in Modern America.* New York: Routledge, 2001.

Stalhurt, R. W. "Concentrations of Urinary Phthalate Metabolites Are Associated with Increased Waist Circumference and Insulin Resistance in Adult U.S. Males." NCBI Pubmed. June 2007. Department of Community and Preventive Medicine, University of Rochester School of Medicine and Dentistry, Rochester, NY. http://www.ncbi.nlm.nih.gov/pubmed/17589594?ordinalpos=1&itool=EntrezSystem2.PEntrez.Pubmed.Pubmed_ResultsPanel.Pubmed_RVDocSum (accessed. 15 August 2008).

California State Board of Barbering. *Health and Safety for Hair Care and Beauty Professionals.* Berkeley: Labor Occupational Health Program, Center for Occupational and Environmental Health, 1993.

Sathyanarayana, Sheela, Catherine J. Karr, Paula Lozano, Elizabeth Brown, Antonia M. Calafat, Fan Liu, and Shanna H. Swan. "Baby Care Products: Possible Sources of Infant Phthalate Exposure." *Pediatrics* 121(2) (February 2008): e260–e268. http://pediatrics.aappublications.org/cgi/content/full/121/2/e260 (accessed 3 June 2009).

Swan, Shanna H., Katharina M. Main, Fan Liu, Sara L. Stewart, Robin L. Kruse, Antonia M. Calafat, Catherine S. Mao, J. Bruce Redmon, Christine L. Ternand, Shannon Sullivan, J. Lynn Teague, and the Study for Future Families Research Team. "Decrease in Anogenital Distance Among Male Infants with Prenatal Phthalate Exposure." *Environmental Health Perspectives* 113, no. 8 (August 2005): 1056–61. www.ehponline.org/members/2005/8100/8100.html

Thompson, J. Kevin. *Exacting Beauty: Theory, Assessment, and Treatment of Body Image.* Washington, DC: American Psychological Association, 1999.

Timbrell, John A. *The Poison Paradox: Chemicals as Friends and Foes.* Oxford and New York: Oxford University Press, 2005.

United States Code, Title 21, *Food and Drugs.* Chapter 9: Federal Food, Drug, and Cosmetic Act. Pub. L. 361–364. January 2007.

U.S. Food and Drug Administration. Center for Food Safety and Applied Nutrition /Office of Cosmetics and Colors. "Phthalates and Cosmetic Products." Washington, DC: Department of Health and Human Services, 2008.

U.S. Food and Drug Administration. Center for Food Safety and Applied Nutrition /Office of Cosmetics and Colors. "FDA Authority Over Cosmetics." Washington, DC: Department of Health and Human Services, 2005.

Vinikas, Vincent. *Soft Soap, Hard Sell: American Hygiene in an Age of Advertisement.* Ames: Iowa State University Press, 1992.

Williams, Rose Marie. "Cosmetic Chemicals and Safer Alternatives." *Townsend Letter,* February/March 2004.

Websites

PubMed: www.ncbi.nlm.nih.gov/pubmed

Chemidex: www.chemidex.com

U.S. Department of Health and Human Services: http://hhs.gov

Index

The Index contains only those ingredients discussed in the text.